Luiz Eduardo Almeida
Marília Nalon Pereira

Integration Seminar: humanization in focus

Luiz Eduardo Almeida
Marília Nalon Pereira

Integration Seminar: humanization in focus

Descriptive analysis of a course

ScienciaScripts

Imprint

Cover image: www.ingimage.com

This book is a translation from the original published under ISBN 978-3-330-77327-1.

Publisher:
Sciencia Scripts
is a trademark of
Dodo Books Indian Ocean Ltd. and OmniScriptum S.R.L publishing group

120 High Road, East Finchley, London, N2 9ED, United Kingdom
Str. Armeneasca 28/1, office 1, Chisinau MD-2012, Republic of Moldova, Europe
Managing Directors: Ieva Konstantinova, Victoria Ursu
info@omniscriptum.com

Printed at: see last page
ISBN: 978-620-8-64667-7

SUMMARY

DEDICATORY

TO GOD,

for enabling life and relationships...

*To my **PARENTS**, **CELSO** and **GRACINHA**,*

for his example of courage and dedication.

For teaching me the meaning of the word family.

I thank you for everything you have done, do and will do for me.

I love you!!!

*To my **BROTHERS**, **ADRIANA**, **CELSO**, **RONALDO**, **PEDRO** and **LUCIANA**,*

friends, advisors and fighters.

Thank you for your support and encouragement, which make me stronger and more confident.

I always want to be close to you...

*To my advisor, **PROFESSOR MARILIA NALON PEREIRA**, for her example as a human being and educator.*

Thank you for making me see a new, more humane dentistry.

I can say that together we are strong and together we are unbeatable...

ACKNOWLEDGMENTS

There are certainly many examples to follow. I think that giving thanks is not just remembering a few names or places, but recognizing the importance they have had in my life.

Therefore, I would like to thank the friends who attended the Master's Degree in Clinical Dentistry at the Faculty of Dentistry, UFJF, the Professors and the Staff. Please know that you have brought a special meaning to my way of life.

I would also like to thank my everlasting friends from the secretariat, Bernadete (for the warm hugs I received), Flàvia (for her transparency) and Wanessa (for her availability). I couldn't forget my friend and Prof. Dr. Antônio Màrcio and Silvânia, who were fundamental in this important journey of my life. I also remember Prof. Dr. Karina. Karina who welcomed my work.

Thank you for existing and for being part of this story.

"The value of things is not in how long they last, but in how intensely they happen.

That's why there are unforgettable moments,

inexplicable things

and incomparable people".

Fernando Pessoa

ALMEIDA, L. E. **Descriptive analysis of the course "Seminar to Raise Awareness of the Importance of Reception and Humanized Approach": an integration between the School of Dentistry of the Federal University of Juiz de Fora and the National Program for Reorientation of Professional Training in Health (Pró- Saùde)**. Juiz de Fora (MG), 2010. 239f. Dissertation (Stricto Sensu Postgraduate Program - Master's Degree in Clinical Dentistry) - School of Dentistry, Federal University of Juiz de Fora.

SUMMARY

To the detriment of scientific and therapeutic medicine, there is much discussion about a humanized, integral and preventive dental practice. After all, health doesn't simply refer to the absence of disease - biological, social and psycho-affective factors are taken into account. In contrast to this reality, there is the enormous lethargy of faculties in updating their archaic curricula and offering teaching that is in tune with new knowledge and the real needs of the Brazilian population. As a result, higher education institutions need to pay more attention to the training of health professionals, ensuring that students are qualified to practise social dentistry, with a generalist, humanist, critical and reflective outlook, with an entrepreneurial and innovative spirit, based on the ethical and legal principles of the profession. With these questions in mind, this study was proposed based on the importance of introducing humanistic concepts to the training of dental surgeons. This is a qualitative, cross-sectional, descriptive and exploratory study. The experience of the subject "Seminar to Raise Awareness of the Importance of Reception and a Humanized Approach", offered to the second semester, which is part of the new academic curriculum of the School of Dentistry at the Federal University of Juiz de Fora, through the institution's partnership with the National Program for the Reorientation of Professional Training in Health, Pró-Saùde, was presented. The theoretical approach to humanistic concepts was based on lectures, the contents of which were: The health-disease process and its dimensions; Caries and periodontal diseases: a holistic perception; Humanization of dental care; The SUS in higher education (Pró-Saùde); Notions of bioethics; Management in Dentistry: how to plan, develop and evaluate an educational-preventive activity. It should also be noted that practical opportunities were provided for the concepts covered through the "Integrated Clinic in Primary Care". Through this experience, it can be concluded that this study served as an important step towards valuing the social aspect of dentistry, which required a pedagogical practice geared towards the emerging paradigms of education, which guide the teaching-learning process, This means viewing the student as a complete being, capable of producing knowledge, transforming reality and, when entering the world of work, perceiving their patient as a human being with biological, social and psycho-affective needs, which need to be met in a holistic way.

Keywords: Humanization of Care; Higher Education; Health Professionals.

1 INTRODUCTION

"... humanizing is the art of developing our senses and making this a strong ally in dental care, guaranteeing the patient humanized care, as they deserve (ALMEIDA, 2009, p.120)

1 INTRODUCTION

The term humanization has recurred in scientific publications on health care and assistance, whether related to hospitalization, ethics, technology, health policies, teaching or the relationship between health professionals and the person who seeks their services - after all, the process of humanization must go through the whole of society.

At a time when the theme of humanization occupies an important place in contemporary debates on training and health work, it is urgent that the concept of "humanization" be re-evaluated and criticized. This urgency can be seen in the trivialization and fragmentation with which the topic has been treated in some of the biomedical and health literature: sometimes it appears as a notion aimed at alleviating a capitalist and exclusionary medical practice; sometimes as the search for a lost moral essence; sometimes as a simple negative perception of reality; sometimes as an appreciation of social rights - in other words, the fragmented development of humanistic concepts puts the motivations of the humanizing movement on different and even conflicting paths, weakening and even inhibiting its action (PUCCINI and CECILIO, 2004; BENEVIDES and PASSOS, 2005a).

Within these questions, Almeida, 2009, p.119-120, explained:

"[...] I remember as if it were today how strange I felt about the word humanization: after all, if I am a human being, the patient is the same [...] After all, what is humanization? I believe that humanized care is care in which the patient receives from me, the academic, comprehensive care for their real needs: biological, social and psycho-affective [...] I would add that in order to humanize a relationship we have to sharpen our senses. Sight, smell, taste, touch and hearing are not enough as physiological resources, in fact we have to use them as allies within the dental clinic. Sight is not just seeing the patient, but assessing him clinically: his face is in a lot of pain, he looks insecure? Wouldn't touch be a good measure to establish a link between patient and professional [...] And so the other senses follow [...] I conclude that humanizing is the art of developing our senses and making them a strong ally in dental care, guaranteeing the patient the humanized care they deserve."

Critics of the humanizing proposals in the field of health denounce the fact that the initiatives underway are often reduced to changes that do not effectively call into question the established models of care and management (BENEVIDES and PASSOS, 2005b). However, the issue has become so important that a National Humanization Policy (PNH) has even been created within the Ministry of Health (BRASIL, 2004a). Even so, there is no way of guaranteeing a national policy for the humanization of health without confronting the issue of humanism in the contemporary world.

Regardless of concepts and designations, it can be said that when it comes to humanization, there seems to be a consensus that the central issue is the subject, the person seeking the health service, characterizing humanized care as that which is personalized. Furthermore, any health care implies a relationship between people, which in this case is between the professional and the person receiving the care. The fact that the health professional is also considered a subject establishes a subject-subject relationship, which will allow this to be classified as

interaction as humanized is the quality of the relationship (PESSINI et al., 2003).

So, one might ask, what is the point of debating humanization if it doesn't actually bring about concrete changes in the practice of health services and in the quality of services offered to the population? It's obvious that the answer lies in the need and challenge to change the way we do things, work and produce health (BENEVIDES and PASSOS, 2005b).

Nevertheless, the Ministry of Health is convinced that the investment in the physical network, technology and supplies is in vain if health professionals don't put their faith in the Unified Health System (SUS) (BRASIL, 2007).

This non-humanized practice of health professionals is largely due to the mismatch between what is taught in higher education institutions (HEIs) and the real needs of the Brazilian population. In fact, HEIs must take on board their role of reflecting on what they are producing and reproducing as a transforming element with a commitment to society (ALMEIDA, 2009).

The National Curriculum Guidelines (DCN) for Undergraduate Dentistry Courses, defined by the National Education Council of the Ministry of Education, provide for an educational process that considers curriculum integration as a strategy for training a generalist, **humanist**, critical and reflective professional to work at all levels of health care, based on technical and scientific rigor (BRASIL, 2002).

Faced with this curricular change, we can't count on a spontaneous change in the way HEIs think. With this in mind, the Ministry of Health, through the Secretariat for Work Management and Health Education (SGTES) and the Ministry of Education, through the Secretariat of Higher Education (SESu) and the National Institute of Educational Studies and Research Anisio Teixeira (INEP), launched the National Program for the Reorientation of Professional Training in Health (Pró-Saùde) in November 2005 (BRASIL, 2007).

Thus, Pró-Saùde, which conceives the need for health workers to be central to the promotion, protection and recovery of health and the production of care, recognizes the need to transform the professional training process. To this end, it recognizes and focuses on the need for teaching-service integration, as well as the consequent inclusion of students in the real scenario of practice, with an emphasis on primary care, from the very beginning of their training (BRASIL, 2007).

The construction of pedagogical practices in higher education committed to humanization requires as a challenge the design of new humanized pedagogical projects, demanded by contemporary society in the field of Dentistry (MOYSÉS, 2003). Deslandes, 2005, adds that investing in the training of professionals with this new outlook, from their first experiences of socialization and school life, is an important strategy, the sustainability of which is based on the dissemination of counter-hegemonic ideological mechanisms and alliances that guarantee adherence and continuous renewal of the proposal.

Therefore, in order for there to be a real introduction not only of the concepts of humanization, but also the awakening of a humanizing awareness and experience in dental practice, we need to think about a participatory training process in search of the construction of new meanings in favour of the defence of life, which meets the new challenges of Brazilian dentistry and the social demands for more oral health. It concludes that Humanization in Health must be imperative.

From this perspective, this study proposes a strategy to analyze the pedagogical content of the subject "Seminar to Raise Awareness of the Importance of Reception and a Humanized Approach", which is part of the curriculum of the Dentistry course at the Federal University of Juiz de Fora, Its sustainability is based on the dissemination of counter-hegemonic ideological mechanisms and alliances that guarantee adherence and renewal in the way of thinking and, above all, acting in the field of dental work - which requires deep reflection and changes in professional training.

2 THEORETICAL FOUNDATIONS

"Any research, on whatever scale, will involve reading what other people have written about your area of interest, gathering information to support or refute these arguments and writing up your conclusions (BELL, 2008, p.57).

2 THEORETICAL FOUNDATIONS

2.1 PRACTICE AND PROFESSIONAL TRAINING IN DENTISTRY IN BRAZIL

2.1.1 Contextualizing dental practice: to understand the present, it is necessary to know the past

Currently, there is a lot of discussion about dental practice - a deeper understanding of this subject, however, requires an understanding of the historical evolution of the paradigms of medical practice, since dentistry is a regionalized expression of that practice (ALMEIDA, 2009).

This evolution, directly related to political, social and economic issues in society and, above all, adjusted to capitalist impositions, is based on three paradigms: sanitarism; scientific, technicist or positivist (Flexnerian) medicine; and community (promotional) medicine (BARROS, 1996; CARVALHO and KRIGER, 2006; BUSS, 2000; MENEZES and LORETTO, 2006; PAIM, 2004; ROSA and LABATE, 2005; SANTOS and WESTPHAL, 1999).

In the 19th century, the field of health consisted of empirical, non-specialized medical practice. Despite its simplicity, the health movement that existed at the time managed to influence the health situation in many cities around the world. Its successes contributed to creating the first golden age of public health. The work, however, was organized in the form of a campaign, along military lines, with the characteristic authoritarianism. The ability to communicate and mobilize the population was almost zero. Actions were not made available, they were imposed; the main objective was to fight disease and, above all, to get good results. With the arrival of Enlightenment ideas, which believed in the primacy of intelligence and reason, critical thinking developed to oppose current sanitary practices, emphasizing the importance of scientific knowledge (BARROS, 1996; CARVALHO and KRIGER, 2006; BUSS, 2000; MENEZES and LORETTO, 2006; PAIM, 2004; ROSA and LABATE, 2005; SANTOS and WESTPHAL, 1999).

Scientific medicine emerged during the formative period of monopoly capitalism, between the end of the 19th century and the beginning of the 20th century. This was a time of tacit acceptance of reformist movements aimed at creating a modern state, governed by the laws of science and designed to exercise forms of social control that could resolve the contradictions generated by industrialization. Thus, the idea of the biological nature of disease took hold in medicine, shifting causal thinking in health from the physical and social environment to concrete pathogens, in other words, disease had only one cause: a germ originating each etiology. This gave rise to the idea that health was simply the absence of disease (BARROS, 1996; CARVALHO and KRIGER, 2006; BUSS,

2000; MENEZES and LORETTO, 2006; PAIM, 2004; ROSA and LABATE, 2005; SANTOS and WESTPHAL, 1999).

In this way, there was and still is an academic effort to change medical education, which until then had been unprepared for new demands and ideas. The new paradigm expresses a set of elements that direct medical practice: curativism, mechanicism, biologicism, individualism, the exclusion of alternative practices, the technification of the medical act, the emphasis on curative medicine, the concentration of resources and specialization. From this moment on, medical practice began to focus on curing individuals who manifested an illness, ushering in the therapeutic era, which has been consolidated and is still in force today (BARROS, 1996; CARVALHO and KRIGER, 2006; BUSS, 2000; MENEZES and LORETTO, 2006; PAIM, 2004; ROSA and LABATE, 2005; SANTOS and WESTPHAL, 1999).

In dentistry, there is a clear scientific influence, which is still reflected in a technical dental practice aimed at patients with greater purchasing power or from favored social classes, thus configuring the model of the liberal professional in dentistry, meaning that the professional is prepared to offer certain types of work in exchange for a certain payment (ALMEIDA, 2009). However, according to Valença, 1998, there is a clear contradiction between the desire for profit of a fundamentally liberal professional class and the purchasing power of large sections of the population. In addition, Freitas, 2001, p.78, adds: *"the status of dentists who dedicate themselves to primary care and public service is lower than that of their own colleagues"*.

In the same vein, Pinto, 2000, p.2, puts forward the idea that dental practice is based on a perverse model of organization, which often ends up *"concentrating the supply of services among middle- and high-income groups, resulting in a narrowing of the scope of technological advances that end up benefiting only the most economically advantaged sectors of the population"*. Moreira et al., 2007, 1388, describes the worsening of social exclusion brought about by scientific dental practice:

"/.../ precarious living conditions make it difficult to prioritize health care. Although they suffer from dental pain, going to the dentist is perceived as a luxury, not a citizen's right. Difficult access to services and poor quality restorations favor tooth extraction as the most effective solution. The deterioration of oral health is lamented by residents who seek help from popular clinics, politicians and healers. The experience of dental disease differs according to class, leaves oral marks of inequality and damages self-esteem and social inclusion. "Treating" the teeth of inequality in this context requires a deeper understanding of the social determinants of health, reducing injustices in access to quality services, removing demoralizing stigmas and strengthening the community's voice in the face of the structural forces that affect their lives."

Almeida, 2009, p.135, adds:

"[...] with the intense appreciation of appearance in society, poor oral health further amplifies existing social inequalities, increasing discrimination and social exclusion. After all, tooth loss causes a deep

loss of self-esteem and insecurity in personal and work relationships, resulting in isolation, rejection and loss of opportunities."

Thus, historically, dental professionals have organized themselves around the care of small population groups, in other words, around the enrolled clientele who sought dental care (BOTAZZO, 2000). Furthermore, as Botazzo (2000) points out, many candidates for the title of dental surgeon seek only to obtain prestige and social ascension. Based on this reality, dentition can be an expression of unequal life paths (GOFFMAN, 1988; RODRIGUES, 1979; WOLF, 1998).

Botazzo, 2000, p.21, within a critical perception, characterizes the

Dentistry as *"a discipline that claims to name the mouth as its object and exercises its dominion over it"*. He adds that the practice of this discipline is often alienated from its public commitment to health and citizenship. There are several elements to criticize in the profession, including commercialism, elitism and a pronounced taste for the surface of its object.

According to the Final Report of the First National Oral Health Conference (I CNSB), 1986, p.4, the current model of dental practice *"covers the needs of only 5% of the population."* In addition, this report highlights the concentration of professionals in large urban centers, including the Public Services located there, the limited use of elementary and middle-level auxiliary personnel, the almost inexpressive use, in a systematized way, of preventive methods of a collective nature, the lack of democratization of knowledge and information on oral health to the population, the tendency to value specialty over general practice, the proliferation of dental schools, with a drop in the level of teaching and, finally, the inadequacy of the trained professional to the needs of the community and the social reality in which they live (BRASIL, 1086a).

The final document of the II National Oral Health Conference, 1993, p.4, reaffirms the points made at the I CNSB, interpreting that the oral health model in force in Brazil is characterized by:

"[...] It has an extremely limited capacity to respond to the needs of the Brazilian population, it is ineffective in intervening in the prevalence of oral diseases that plague the country, it is elitist, uncoordinated, diffuse, individualistic, mutilating, iatrogenic, high cost, low social impact and disconnected from the epidemiological and social reality of the nation."

In this context, Weyne, 1999, p.5, points out that *"dentistry must broaden its ethical commitments to society and the social"*, so that people can live healthy lives. Therefore, we need to think about changing the traditional form of treatment centered on the disease, which has been hegemonic until now, to another type of professional, whose ideology is the prevention of diseases and the promotion of health.

Santos, 1989, p.22, reported that:

"Logical positivism represents [...] the apogee of the dogmatization of science, that is, of a conception of science that sees it as the privileged apparatus for representing the world, with no other

foundations than the basic propositions about the coincidence between the univocal language of science and immediate experience or observation, with no other limits than those resulting from the stage of development of experimental or logical-deductive instruments."

It is true that the gains brought about by modern science cannot be dismissed, but, according to Matos, 2006, some reflections become fundamental:

"What has science actually done for the essential problems of humanity, such as hunger, social inequalities, poverty and war? Which problems does it address and which does it exclude because they don't fit into its method, because they don't confer scientific status or power; because they don't have instrumental, technical or financial return purposes for industries? And have the ethical problems inherent in research and its practical purposes been given the scientific space they deserve, or does everyone get their fair share? Is it up to scientists to do the research, while it's up to politicians and businessmen to decide the fate of the product of science? In short, these are questions that epistemology can no longer postpone; they prompt immediate reflection in the direction of a more just and humane society." (MATOS, 2006, p.137)

Based on the underlying criticisms of modern science, which according to Santos, 1989, p.11, is plunged into a deep crisis, this is a time of transition between modern science and a new paradigm that the author calls *"postmodern science"*. The same author adds that in order to sustain itself, post-modern science has to emerge from a double epistemological rupture. The first is the rupture with common sense and the second, which is still in process, is the rupture with the unconditional hegemony of modern science, in other words, a paradigm that has progressively shaped the world through science and technology, which demands distance and estrangement between subject and object; which is guided by the principles of instrumental rationality, but which is not responsible for the possible irrationality of the technical applications it produces; a paradigm that marginalizes other forms of knowledge (religious, artistic, literary, mythical, poetic and political) in society; that separates theory from practice, science from ethics; in short, a paradigm that produces a discourse that purports to be rigorous and objective, but is disenchanted, sad and lacking in imagination (SANTOS, 1989).

Nevertheless, it can be said that, as with sanitarism, scientism is entering a crisis due to growing problems related to inefficiency, ineffectiveness and, above all, the incoherence of this paradigm with the instruments of action of the public health system in force in Brazil: the SUS (ALMEIDA, 2009).

As a result of this and its own structural characteristics, scientific medicine became highly selective and therefore unattainable for the majority of the population, giving way to the community model. In 1986, Brazil held the 8th National Health Conference, whose theme was "Democracy is Health" and which was a forum for fighting for the decentralization of the health system and the implementation of social policies that defended and cared for life. The final report of this Conference laid the foundations for the proposal for the Unified Health System (SUS), the basis of which is the creation process: the expanded concept of health, the need to create public policies to promote it, the imperative of social participation in the construction of the health system and policies and the impossibility of the health sector to respond alone to the transformation of the determinants and conditioning factors to guarantee healthy options for the population (BRASIL, 1986b).

It's worth noting that there is still a great deal of lethargy on the part of undergraduate courses in updating their curricula in line with the new knowledge (WEYNE, 1999). Based on this, the Ministry of Health is convinced that investment in adapting the physical network, technology, medicines and supplies is in vain if health professionals don't bet on the Unified Health System (SUS) - which means reaffirming within higher education institutions the constitutional principles of universality, equity and integrality of the actions established for the SUS (BRASIL, 2007).

Dentistry has the majority of dentists who are not involved in health promotion, protection and recovery and the production of care, which generates the corollary need for transformations in the process of training these professionals, correcting a mismatch between the orientation of training - still scientific - and the principles, guidelines and needs of the SUS (BRASIL, 2007;

CARVALHO and KRIGER, 2006).

Thus, to situate the problem of monitoring inequalities in

health associated with the profile of social vulnerabilities is to understand the need for dialog between different disciplines and theoretical and methodological affiliations. Only from this interdisciplinary perspective is it possible to build new and significant information bases for the design and implomontation of hoalth polioioo oapablo of rcoponding to thc challcngc of social vulnerabilities.

social inequalities (MAGALHAES, 2007).

It can be concluded, according to Werneck and Lucas, 1996, that in order to be effective

of this type of action, it is important to highlight two aspects:

"[...] it is believed that the key to the success of a dentistry course is a qualified teaching staff committed to its mission. When selecting teachers, technical qualifications and a commitment to providing health services should be taken into account; b) although the public sector is the main employer of dental surgeons and professional training should be geared to occupational and epidemiological profiles, there is still a lack of coordination between dental schools and oral health services'.

2.1.2 The dental training model

In general terms, professional training is a fundamental factor in improving the health system and, consequently, people's quality of life, since it is human resources, through their status as subjects of the work process, that give different characteristics to each health service produced (NARVAI, 1999).

Dental education has been based on a model of dentistry that has not been effective in generating health, either for the social majority or for the elites. One of the causes of this problem is the exclusionary nature of the model practiced, which focuses on market logic, available to those with purchasing power, thus excluding the social majority (PÉRET, 2005).

In addition, public policies have not provided benefits in the dental field for this social class, which has aggravated the exclusionary nature. On the other hand, the model practiced has also shown that, even in the most privileged segments of the population, who enjoy the best and most sophisticated restorative equipment and materials, it has not been possible to achieve a consistent increase in oral health levels (WEYNE, 1999).

Knowledge of the processes relating to the evolution of education and practice in the health sector needs to be understood within a political context. In Marcos' view, 1984, the model of practice, the training of human resources, the production of knowledge and its distribution reflect society's economic mode of production and the struggle between social forces.

In light of the above, many criticisms are currently being leveled at the profile of dental surgeons graduating from Brazilian universities. However, according to Almeida, 2009, before deciding on the type of university you want to build, you need to think about the type of professional you want to develop.

According to Araùjo, 2006, p.3, the training of professionals in dental schools in Brazil must be in direct interface with the real oral health needs of the population and inserted in the paradigm of public health policy and the principles of the Unified Health System:

"The relationship between health and education concerns the adaptation of professionals to the social needs of the population. This relationship will be achieved through effective interaction between the training of health professionals, the health services of the SUS and the communities, constituting an important strategy for promoting the necessary changes in academic training".

It is worth emphasizing that training processes must take into account the rapid pace of knowledge evolution, changes in the health work process, transformations in demographic and epidemiological aspects, with a view to balancing technical excellence and social relevance. (BRASIL, 2007). In addition, according to Werneck and Lucas, 1996, p.15, these desired transformations require higher education institutions to *"have an enormous need to re-see, re-think and re-create their practices".*

Almeida, 2009, p.128, contextualizes the need for intervention in the training process in dentistry:

"[...to shift the axis of training, which is still centered on the biological approach, towards more contextualized training, which takes into account the social, economic and cultural dimensions of the health/disease process - thus taking into account the formation of a qualified professional for the practice of social dentistry, with a generalist, humanist, critical and reflective vision, with an entrepreneurial and innovative spirit, capable of acting in a multi-professional, interdisciplinary and trans-disciplinary manner, with productivity at the levels of promotion, prevention, treatment and rehabilitation at all levels of health care based on technical-scientific rigor, knowing and

understanding the social reality in order to intervene in the oral health problems of the population, based on the ethical and legal principles of the profession'

According to Carli, 2007, pp.31-32:

"Regarding the traditional training of the Brazilian dental surgeon, it can be said that its most important bias, that is, the disjunctive paradigm, when applied to curricula and disciplines, after successive reforms of a Flexnerian nature, emphasized cognitive and instrumental dominance, with some of the following consequences: mechanicism, biologicism, individual assistance, early specialization, technification of the medical-dental act, emphasis on curative medicine/dentistry."

Within this logic, Kriger, 2005, stated that traditional training in

health, based on disciplinary organization and specialties, leads to the fragmented study of the health problems of people and societies, and consequently leads to the formation of specialists who can no longer deal with totalities or complex realities.

With the increase in the number of colleges in the country over the last two decades, the quality of oral health has not improved. This is because the current teaching model is incapable of providing health care for a large part of the population. University education is very deficient in relation to subjects that deal with social and preventive aspects, often leading to a lack of interest on the part of future professionals (AMARAL, 1991). According to studies by Harrison and Wong, 2003, the university must take on the role of reflecting on what it is producing and reproducing as a transforming element and commitment to society.

In a didactic way, Weyne, 1999, explained the fragility of dental training centered on surgical-restorative foundations, using caries and periodontal diseases as examples, showing the immense fragility of assessing the activity and severity of these diseases based solely on an analysis of the anatomical and morphological characteristics of their lesions - it is clear the failure of simplistic conceptions, in which treatment involved only restoring the tooth or extracting it - which led to new visions of treatment being proposed. Thus, dentistry curricula, which have always focused on treatment, must undergo permanent renewal, intense updating and systematic conceptual change (ALMEIDA, 2009).

Busato et al., 2001, p. 335, stated that no model is better than prevention. Prevention, which means educating for health: *"Maximum Prevention... Maximum Preservation... Minimal Intervention. No professional training policy in dentistry can ignore these concepts".*

Finally, according to Luzuriaga, 1960, p.308:

"[...] vocational education must have a very close relationship both with the scientific and technical progress of the time and with the economic life of the country or region, and cannot therefore be disconnected from the larger context."

In this sense, adapting the academic curriculum to the country's epidemiological, social and economic reality has become an extremely important aspect of dental surgeon training (PINTO, 2000).

2.1.3 Curricular aspects: National Curriculum Guidelines

Law 9394/1996 (Lei de Diretrizes e Bases da Educaçao) replaced the minimum curriculum with curricular guidelines, and the National Education Council approved the National Curricular Guidelines (DCN) for health courses between 2001 and 2002 (Resoluçâo CNE/CES, de 19 de fevereiro de 2002 - DCN do Curso de Graduaçâo em Odontologia) (BRASIL, 2002).

The Guidelines seek to advance the organization of the curricula of higher education courses in the health area, overcoming "the old conceptions of curricular grids, often used as mere instruments for transmitting knowledge and information". They reinforce the articulation between Higher Education and Health, "aiming at the general and specific training of graduates/professionals with an emphasis on health promotion, prevention, recovery and rehabilitation" and, in this way, "the concept of health and the principles and guidelines of the Unified Health System (SUS) are fundamental elements to be emphasized in this articulation" (BRASIL, 2001).

The DCN defines the principles, foundations, conditions and procedures for the training of dental surgeons:

"The profile of the graduate/professional must be generalist, humanist, critical and reflective, to work at all levels of health care, based on technical and scientific rigor. They must be trained to carry out activities relating to the oral health of the population, based on ethical and legal principles and an understanding of the social, cultural and economic reality of their environment, directing their work towards transforming reality for the benefit of society" (BRASIL, 2002, p. 10).

Kriger, 2005, defined this professional with a generalist profile as follows: they must understand the logic of the health-disease process, understand the cycle of

life, have an understanding of oral diseases (relationship with other diseases), build a reasoning process for clinical intervention, act on the dynamics of life and the community, intervene on the family, have the competence to make a diagnosis, make good therapy, a humane and ethical approach, be resolutive. They must combine clinical competence with social responsibility.

The DCN also sets out the general and specific competences and skills that should result from the professional training of dental surgeons. The general skills require: health care, decision-making, communication, leadership, administration and management, as well as continuing education (BRASIL, 2002).

Among the specific skills to be developed are those required to collect, observe and interpret data for the construction of a diagnosis; identify prevalent oral and maxillofacial conditions; develop logical reasoning and critical analysis in clinical conduct; propose and execute appropriate treatment plans; carry out health promotion and maintenance; communicate with patients, health professionals and the community in general, within ethical and legal precepts; work in interdisciplinary teams and act as a health promotion agent; plan and administer collective health services; monitor and incorporate technological innovations (IT, new materials, biotechnology) in the exercise of the profession (BRASIL, 2002).

Bearing in mind that the Resolution on the DCN has general, wide-ranging characteristics and a great deal of flexibility, the Brazilian Dental Education Association (ABENO) drew up some recommendations for the implementation of these Guidelines, disseminating them to courses and at a meeting held in parallel with the 20th International Dental Congress of São Paulo, promoted by the São Paulo Dental Surgeons Association in January 2002.

(ABENO, 2002).

Bezerra and Paula, 2003, p. 13-14, reported the following conclusions from their study

work on the curricular structure of dentistry courses in Brazil:

"The curricula express a range of variations in the composition of their respective workloads, with the prominent treatment given to technical training and the separation between basic and vocational training areas in the formally structured curricula being clear points of agreement; the treatment given to the areas of Collective Health and Ethics and Citizenship is quite disparate, depending on the profile that each course intends to give its students; the introduction of new areas of knowledge is incipient, which denotes the lack of attention paid to the subject by the administration of the courses; there is a need to reorient the courses to the new Curricular Guidelines".

According to Pizzatto et al., 2004, the national scene is made up of courses and courses in dentistry. Within this context, one comes across colleges - unfortunately, they are still a minority - which, even before the entry into force of the Law of Guidelines and Bases, had already woken up to the need to reformulate the current curriculum, directing efforts towards the training of a professional able to face the real needs of the population.

Dental teaching has been based on technical content strongly rooted in the outpatient clinic of dental schools and the social approach to health problems is not a topic frequently discussed among students and teachers (MATOS and TOMITA, 2005).

According to interviews conducted by Secco and Pereira, 2004, some coordinators of dentistry courses consider that the lack of a more politicized training in the area, which considers the challenges of the Brazilian reality and problematizes the professional imaginary, is reproduced in the courses, making it difficult to participate in public health care policies.

The necessary changes must begin in professional training and in the worldview reproduced within the academies, because it is certainly in these spaces that the possibilities for the future employability of dental surgeons and their social relevance also begin. The great dilemma in dealing with issues like this is that every change brings "discomfort" (MOYSÉS, 2004).

According to Struchiner, Vieira and Ricciardi, 2005, the curriculum should promote a rapprochement between basic scientific concepts and clinical practice, which should emphasize the solution of the population's problems, from a realistic perspective.

It is worth noting that through the curriculum structure, the courses and faculties

determine the profile of future professionals. For higher education in the health area, it is recommended that future professionals should be able to work with "quality, efficiency and resolution in the Unified Health System (SUS)" (BRASIL, 2001).

Finally, Lucietto, 2005, p.65:

"Attention is drawn to the fact that these guidelines have taken into account both the concept of health and the principles of the Unified Health System, and point to it as one of the essential aspects for training in dentistry, stipulating that "the training of dental surgeons should take into account the health system in force in the country, comprehensive health care in a regionalized and hierarchical system of reference and counter-reference, and teamwork". In this way, the inclusion of students in public services plays a fundamental role in the process. The establishment of these guidelines is triggering curricular reform processes in all the country's dentistry courses. In this sense, there are expectations regarding the operationalization of the intended changes and also the results of these guidelines on the profile of future dental surgeons, with regard to their competences/qualifications to work adequately within the scope of the Unified Health System. At the very least, they point to the fact that there has been a rapprochement between the Ministries of Health and Education, which is indispensable for the training of human resources in health in the current Brazilian situation'.

2.1.4 National Program for the Reorientation of Professional Training in Health (Pro-Health): a new proposal for the training of human resources in higher education in health

According to Almeida, 2009, p.13:

"The Unified Health System effectively constitutes a job market for health professionals, both in public and contracted services, and represents a new standard of practice that demands a reorientation of training - although this fact has not yet been realized by a large part of academia."

According to Zanetti, 2001, work processes in public services are more complex than those in private practice. As such, in addition to most of the skills required of dentists working in the service market, others are also required in order to ensure qualified public practice.

As pointed out earlier, one of SUS's attributions in the 1988 Federal Constitution is to *"organize the training of human resources in the health area"* (1988 Federal Constitution, art. 200, item III). However, according to Morita and Kriger, 2004, although this precept exists, it has not been implemented as an institutional practice. The authors, p.17, state that:

"[...] previous efforts to integrate the teaching-learning process of the dental student into the service network, until then, had little sustainability, since they happened more because of the ideological adherence of teachers and students.

The current National Curriculum Guidelines for Dentistry Courses value the inclusion of students in the Unified Health System. In this sense, Morita and Kriger, 2004, p.18, based on the guidelines, state that *"to work in the SUS with quality and meet the needs of the population, it is necessary to be a technically competent generalist professional with social sensitivity".*

To the detriment of this, Almeida, 2009, p.13, states:

"It can also be seen that scientific research has been predominantly focused on specialized aspects usually linked to high technology, when in reality, without detriment to that, it is necessary to deepen studies and research in the field of basic care that allow the most relevant aspects to be addressed with effectiveness, quality and resolubility."

In the midst of building a health system based on the principles of integrality, equity and universality, it is essential to train professionals with a critical spirit, who are capable of reflecting and acting in the society in which they are inserted (ALMEIDA, 2009). In this sense, it is necessary to *"realize that social reality is not a mass of fragmented and disconnected facts, but is complex, contradictory, comprising relationships, processes and structures that are not always visible"* (IYDA, 1998, p.138). Thus, the facts must be unraveled so that reality can be captured in its totality, that is, in movement and, more than that, the solution to its contradictions must be sought, creating a new reality (IYDA, 1998).

Health professionals must have technical, communicative, social and organizational skills, the ability to take responsibility for patient care and attention, the ability to constantly reflect on and evaluate the world of work, new ethical and professional commitments and new attitudes as citizens. In other words, health professionals are expected to act more adequately in today's society, with a view to the world of tomorrow (NORONHA, 2002).

It should be noted that many academic institutions' own services follow their own internal logic, which is more linked to the demands of research and teaching than to the real demands of offering referrals and counter-referrals to the SUS network (ALMEIDA, 2009). In this sense, it must be assumed that one cannot depend on a spontaneous transformation of public academic institutions in the direction indicated by the SUS (BRASIL, 2007). For this reason, playing an inductive role is extremely important, in order to give direction to the process of change and facilitate the achievement of the proposed objectives in the search for more equitable and quality health care (BRASIL, 2007).

In order to reverse this situation, the National Program for the Reorientation of Professional Training in Health, Pró-Saùde, was presented on November 3, 2005, with the signing of an Interministerial Ordinance by the Ministry of Health and the Ministry of Education (BRASIL, 2007).

Pró-Saùde, an expanded development of a previous proposal aimed only at medical courses

(PROMED), is, along with a number of other initiatives, a response to the need to train generalist professionals with a profile to meet the national health policy in the primary care strategy. Pró-saùde presents (BRASIL, p.5, 2007):

"The aim is to intervene in the training process so that undergraduate programs can shift the axis of training - centered on individual care provided in specialized units - to another process in which training is attuned to social needs, based on the proposal of hierarchical health actions. In addition, training should take into account the social, economic and cultural dimensions of the population, equipping professionals to address the determinants of both components of the population's health-disease binomial in the community at all levels of the system."

The design of the proposal provided for the participation of both training institutions - with courses in dentistry, medicine and nursing - and the municipal management of the health system, making both sectors jointly responsible and highlighting the involvement of each from the perspective of strengthening and improving the health actions to be carried out within the Unified Health System - defining it as the priority setting for the development of the teaching-learning process (BRASIL, 2007).

The perspective reinforced in the orientation of the axes and vectors of change focuses on some important questions that should guide the changes: what is the concept of the health-disease process adopted, what are the links between the university and the service, what is the relevance of the knowledge produced to the SUS and what is the commitment of the pedagogical orientation (BRASIL, 2007).

The institutions were selected via a joint call for proposals from the Ministry of Education and the Ministry of Health, and the projects have a development schedule, financial incentive and monitoring by the technical department of the Ministry of Health (BRASIL, 2007). Almeida, 2009, p.14, adds that institutions interested in taking part in the selection process would compete by preparing and presenting a project in line with the program's general criteria:

"Clear possibility of articulation with the health service; Guidance on regulation and referral system; Possibility of sharing budget (School and Service); Integration of the Teaching Hospital into the service network; Clear possibility of articulation with the health service; Indication of evaluation parameters."

According to data from the Secretariat for the Management of Work and Education in Health (SGTES), the National Program for the Reorientation of Professional Training in Health selected 90 courses out of 181 projects submitted for evaluation. Of these 90 courses, 38 are in Medicine, 27 in Nursing and 25 in Dentistry. It is worth noting that the program involves 3 years of financial support for projects that have the potential to transform the training model (BRASIL, 2007).

The Federal University of Juiz de Fora, Almeida, 2009, p.15, reports that:

"[.../ its participation in the program presented its projects (Nursing, Medicine and Dentistry), which

focused on the initiative to bring undergraduate education closer to the real needs of primary care. Notwithstanding this perspective, the Faculty of Dentistry, in general terms, aims to develop its project as a school that is integrated with the public health service and that responds to the concrete needs of the Brazilian population in the training of human resources, in the production of knowledge and in the provision of services, all aspects aimed at building the strengthening of the SUS".

2.2 HUMANIZATION IN HEALTH

2.2.1 Humanism and humanization

In the minds of Hippocrates and Galen, a distinction between medical training and humanistic training would seem strange, because they understood that the doctor was, above all, a man perfected by ethics and knowledge about human nature. For them, the doctor is necessarily a humanist. In Galenism, the organic processes and the affective and cognitive activities of man were seen as part of the same vital system, whose balance was guaranteed to the extent that there was a harmonious coexistence between the soul, the mind and the physiological functions. Thus, medical doctrine understood the body as an instrument of perception and action controlled by desires, values and emotions (PESSOTTI, 1996). Although the Greek philosophers had dealt with the subject, *it* fell to Cicero, a Roman politician and orator who lived in the 104-43 century BC, *"to think up and express the term humanitas to designate the set of actions in caring for human formation. Thus, homo humanus emerges to counter homo barbarus"* (HEIDEGGER, 1979, p.7).

According to Foulquié, 1971, humanism is a moral and intellectual movement that aspires to develop the properly human faculties in man. Human comes from the Latin *humanus*, derived from homo (man).

In relation to the term "human", Foulquié, 1971, also says that, in the sense, it refers to someone who feels a sympathy towards their human brothers and sisters that makes them understanding, benevolent and charitable. Houaiss et al., 2001, p.1555, add that human means one who is kind and educated in the humanities and to humanize is to become benevolent, mild, tolerable, treatable.

According to Lalande (1999, p. 1901), a human *being* is the *"individual being who produces the acts or in whom reside the qualities that are affirmed of him"*; they are beings who, according to their values and needs, produce things and build their own history. In this way, the subject is the being of their own life, and their autonomous capacity for relationships or initiatives is their own (Abbagnano, 2000). The same author adds that everything that belongs to the subject is characterized as subjective.

In the semantic biography of the concept of *humanitas*, two significant stages can be identified. The first is equivalent to clemency as a synonym for mercy, meekness and philanthropy. The second, semantic evolution, took on the concept of the human condition in a double meaning, as a style or way of life superior to that of the barbarians and as the perfection of human nature, which points to a radical opposition between man and animal, between man and things (MELO, 2005).

All the types of humanism that have emerged since then and up to the present presuppose the universal *essence of* man as self-evident. This philosopher is concerned that man does not lose his essence as a social being, that the environment he lives in does not make him inhuman, incapable of perceiving himself and others (HEIDGER, 1979).

In this sense, according to Cruz, 2003, the value placed on individuals' capacity for change and choice is directly influenced by the context in which they live. Their values, beliefs and ideologies can be found through studies of social representations which, according to Jodelet, 2001, are complex phenomena that are always activated in social life, or in the workplace.

Thus, according to Rogers, 1992, humanistic theory seeks to value the goodness in people and in human potential, as part of the therapeutic process, which is understood as liberating the individual, in other words, making them believe that they will be happy and satisfied with life. Social representations, according to Moscovici, 2003, seeks to consider human behavior resulting from intentional integrative action as symbolic behavior, as a product of the processes of communication, social interaction and influence, in the context of group relations, with regard to the orientation of the group to which it belongs.

However, with the flourishing of Cartesian thought, the natural sciences and the scientific spirit in the 17th century, medical knowledge moved away from the philosophy of man and any knowledge that didn't have the empirical basis recognized by science was relegated to limbo. In this way, medical knowledge began to reject everything related to human subjectivity. However, in the second half of the 20th century, science itself began to announce the transience of truths and doctrines, so that medical knowledge has proved precarious in many circumstances involving the recognition and understanding of human references that had been discarded for centuries (PESSOTTI, 1996).

Reflecting on the concept of humanization in health, Campos, 2003, p.124, said: *"Human means 'human', that is, biological, subjective and social [...]. We are this all the time, mixed, inseparable, at the same time"*. It's easy to understand why this theme has emerged with such force: health work processes have become increasingly objectified, technified, specialized and commercialized. Houaiss, 2001, states that scientific and technological development has brought countless benefits, but has the adverse effect of increasing dehumanization, which is conceptualized as the loss of human qualities such as personality, spirituality, dignity and character.

Medical culture has promoted a great deception when it cultivates the image of the professional who is unmoved, always cold, never losing his poise, haughty, above human feelings. This is a serious psychological defense that dehumanizes, replacing the feeling and warmth of human exchanges with the relative value, here absolutized, of technical knowledge. Thus, there has been a lot of talk lately about the humanization of medicine, but it is the health professional who needs to be re-humanized, and this through the sincere and protected acceptance of his or her shortcomings and weaknesses. It is not by changing the environment with colors and music or by training the team in an automated way that humanization will take place, but by seeking self-knowledge, giving professionals the opportunity to deal with their internal realities (BENETTON, 2002, p.96).

According to Pessotti, 1996, p.447, it's not a question of being a humanist, although that is also desirable, but of being, to some extent, a humanist: a connoisseur, albeit a beginner, of what constitutes the essence of what is known as human nature, in other words, the essence of those who create values and attribute meanings and senses to the events and conditions of life. To this end, the great challenge, according to Campos, 2003, p.129, is: *"to bring back together what in the historical process has been separated by technical prescriptions, by the social division of labor and by the rejection of subjectivity"*. This subjectivity carries the potential to reintegrate the complex individual and has become, more than ever, one of the greatest challenges in the field of contemporary work.

In this sense, Lévitas, 1993, in admitting that humanism is in crisis, alludes to the fact that the humanistic crisis in our time undoubtedly has its source in the experience of human inefficiency put on trial by the very abundance of means to act and by the extension of ambitions, which are in line with the thoughts of Jodelet, 2001 and Moscovici, 2003.

Man, as a complex being surrounded by diverse situations, whether it's self-realization or understanding others, seeks to "humanize" which, according to Ferreira, 1999, p.346*, is "to make human, to civilize, to give a human condition"* in his social relations. Thus, adds Rizzotto, 2002, p.197:

"[...] only men are capable of promoting and undergoing a process of humanization, and as a process, this is in constant transformation, suffering the influences of the context in which it occurs".

Pearce, 1996 and Abric, 2000 emphasized the need to return to the context in which social interactions take place, as nothing has meaning outside the context in which activities are carried out, since the context is conceived by the person or partly by the group.

With regard to health services, the concern with humanization in the services provided in the name of health is not new. Toledo, 2007, suggests that the first humanization initiative came about with the hospital building, present in the thoughts and actions of the Persian philosopher Avicenna, who lived between 979 and 1037.

In the West, Europeans only began to address the issue at the end of the 18th century, when they established the guidelines for the creation of a new hospital proposal, called a therapeutic hospital by Michel Focault (TOLEDO, 2007).

Molina, 2002, believes that the Universal Declaration of Human Rights, the humanistic milestone of the 20th century, should occupy a central place in the construction of a paradigm for the humanization of health care and in the training of health professionals. Even in the absence of this paradigm in Brazil, questions and discussions about the humanization of healthcare go back several decades (RIZZOTTO, 2002).

In the 1980s, at the heart of the Health Reform Movement, the current model of care was questioned, centered on the figure of the medical professional, biologicism and curative practices. According to Rizzotto, 2002, p. 197,

"This model, according to critics, was very specialized and expensive, emphasized disease to the detriment of health promotion and prevention and was configured as inhumane in the way it assisted, both through the exaggerated use of technologies and the relationship that was established between health professionals and users of the system".

According to this author, with the results of the Health Reform Movement and the popular struggles that marked the 1970s and 1980s, a new health project emerged for the country, which brought with it the possibility of solving a large part of the problems in this public sector. This project, called SUS - Sistema Único de Saù (Unified Health System), carries within it the principles and guidelines of what could be the great policy for humanizing health care in the country. This project guarantees universal, free and comprehensive access for all Brazilians, and removes its begging character to transform it into a right guaranteed in Article 196 of the 1988 Federal Constitution, in the following wording:

"Health is everyone's right and the duty of the State, guaranteed through social and economic policies aimed at reducing the risk of disease and other illnesses and universal and equal access to actions and services for their promotion, protection and recovery" (BRASIL, 1988 p.88).

Subsequently, in compliance with a constitutional mandate, the public authorities regulated the organization of the health care network based on primary care through federal laws 8080\ 90 and 8142\ 90.

"Primary Care is a set of health actions that encompass promotion, prevention, diagnosis, treatment and rehabilitation. It is developed through the exercise of managerial and health practices, which are democratic and participatory, in the form of teamwork, aimed at the populations of well-defined territories, for which it assumes responsibility. [It is guided by the principles of universality, accessibility, continuity, comprehensiveness, accountability, humanization, linkage and social participation" (BRASIL, 2003, p.89).

Thus, it can be concluded that the Unified Health System, which was established, contemplates, in its idea, the organization of the health care network based on Primary Care, recommending as a philosophy the practice of humanized care. Primary Care, as the Brazilian citizen's gateway to the public health system, includes the humanization of care considering the ambience, and as one of its actions, welcoming the user (SOUSA, 2002).

In 2003, the Ministry of Health proposed the National Humanization Policy (PNH) or Policy for the Humanization of Health Care and Management in the Unified Health System: HumanizaSUS (BRASIL, 2006a).

The National Humanization Policy aims to value the different subjects involved in the health production process: users, workers and managers; fostering the autonomy and protagonism of these subjects; increasing the degree of co-responsibility, the production of health and subjects; establishing bonds of solidarity and collective participation in the management process; identification of health needs; change in the models of care and management in the work process, focusing on the needs of citizens and the production of health; commitment to ambience, improvement of working conditions and care (BRASIL, 2006a).

"Ambience in Health refers to the treatment given to the physical space understood as a social, professional and interpersonal relations space, which should provide welcoming, resolutive and humane care" (BRASIL, 2006a, p.5).

Based on this proposal, Humanization is now defined as a policy and no longer as a program. In this way, it implies being taken as a transversal political guideline insofar as it permeates all actions and instances of implementation, as well as translating principles and ways of operating in all the relationships of the different actors in the Unified Health System (SUS) network. It should also be based on building exchanges of solidarity, committed to the dual task of producing health and producing the subject (BRASIL, 2006a).

The guiding principles of the National Humanization Policy include: increasing the degree of co-responsibility of the different actors that make up the SUS network, implying changes in user care and in the management of work processes; valuing the subjective and social dimension in all care and management practices, strengthening and encouraging integrated processes that promote commitment; guaranteeing the conditions for professionals to work in a dignified manner and participate as co-managers of the system, including strengthening work in multi-professional teams (BRASIL, 2006a).

2.2.2 Professional training in dentistry from a humanistic perspective: a paradigm under construction

It is well known that technicism has directly influenced dental education, which has led to a professional formation focused on mechanicism, biologism, an emphasis on individual assistance, early specialization, the technification of the medical-dental act and an emphasis on curative medicine/dentistry - which characterizes the need for a humanization project in dental education, so changing this training framework has been a major challenge (MOYSÉS, 2004).

When Moysés, 2003, p. 94, refers to a project to humanize dental education, there is a reference to the term humanization as an allusion to the inclusion of the area of "humanities", considering that this has man as its central object of reflection. However, it reflects that biomedical education, with its positivist bias and neutralization of the human experience, minimizes the importance of this area.

Thus, Grant, 2002, p. 47, in presenting the justifications for including the Human Sciences in the compulsory curriculum of medical courses, highlights two aspects that reinforce this humanization project:

"[...] first, to improve communication between doctors and patients; second, to increase understanding of the human condition, helping students to better understand the emotional suffering of patients and, once they understand this pain, that they can better understand the disease."

Lucas, 1995, p.215, points out that school is important in professional training, but that there is a set of values such as those acquired in the family, as well as the impositions of the job market, which dictate its forms of organization and the very form of coexistence and reflection that the professional makes in the exercise of their activities. Thus, in order to talk about training, family, school and work must all be involved, which is why the university cannot be held to such high expectations as it currently is.

In this way, it is pertinent to reinforce the idea that the role of the school in training ethical and humane professionals is limited, since, according to Pessotti, 1996, p. 444, the values assumed by men are born out of their personal experience with the objects, acts and events they experience. Thus:

"The basic question of the human individual's relations with others and with society finds its expression in the system of values internalized by the individual. The system of values accepted by the individual exerts a dominant influence on his social relations" (SCHAFF, 1995, p. 141).

When young people choose a career, they have a personal motivation. They carry values that were built up long before they entered the course and which will be added to their career as they come into contact with new theories, clinical experiences and the examples of their teachers, so that each student will see their values confirmed, denied or altered (PESSOTTI, 1996, p. 446). Thus, according to Lucas, 1995, p. 216, the school enhances certain political-professional attitudes or definitions to the extent that it implements projects that create a climate favorable to the development of certain interests, values and commitments.

For Pessoti, 1996, p. 440, a medical school can contribute to the ethical-humanist formation of students both by offering information on these issues and by providing examples of fidelity to these values. In fact, the example is fundamental because it is not the mere knowledge, even critical knowledge, of the ideas of thinkers or social scientists that will ensure a true humanist formation.

Knowledge only guarantees humanistic information, which cannot be dispensed with, because the more doctors know about the humanistic philosophy of their time and the scientific theories about human thought and behavior, the better they will be able to understand the complexity of man that exists beyond morphology (PESSOTTI, 1996, p.444). Proposing this knowledge, however, comes up against the structural elements of formal education which, more often than not, impose huge barriers to medical teaching.

"Certainly, for the young doctor, what philosophy or the "sciences of man" have to say will seem little more than mere speculation, or even metaphysics, after the uncritical information of the course, after

the organicist objectivity, perhaps inevitable, of medical training. It is not uncommon for them to feel like a fish out of water when they read a text on sociology, psychology, epistemology or the history of science. This strangeness has at least two explanations. The first is very obvious: he hasn't been prepared to accept or understand this type of text. The second is less obvious: thanks to scientism (which prevents true scientific information), it is easy for young doctors to develop an attitude of contempt for areas of knowledge that "don't deal with facts" or that don't lead to precise conclusions" (PESSOTTI, 1996, p. 445).

In the process of professional training, with an ethical-humanist profile in mind, it is therefore essential to provide, highlight, discuss and take advantage of everyday school experiences so that students can experience situations that involve the subjectivity of relationships (MATOS, 2006).

When reflecting on the humanistic training of health professionals, it is necessary to bear in mind, according to Pessotti, 1996, p. 447, that the ability to understand others depends, in the clinic or outside it, on the professional's self-knowledge. Thus:

"[...] any humanistic education program must develop in students an awareness of their own values, of their own humanity. For it is this awareness that will filter information (curricular or otherwise) about the nature and history of man" (PESSOTTI, 1996, p. 447).

In view of this, self-knowledge is the fundamental experience that school education should provide, i.e. students' perception of their own desires, beliefs, shortcomings, defects and qualities. It is from this awareness that health professionals will be built who are able to grow in their interaction with patients, in a welcoming and humane way (MATOS, 2006). This is complemented by Pereira, p.87-88, 2000, who stated that awareness of the de-monopolization of dental knowledge, centered on interdisciplinarity and participatory human relationships, would contribute in leaps and bounds to meaningful learning that is never forgotten, changing the profile of the future professional.

2.2.3 Problematizing methodology: from observation to application in reality

The problematizing methodology aims to increase the student's capacity to become a participant and an agent of social transformation, developing in them the ability to observe the immediate or surrounding reality, detect all available resources and find ways of organizing work and collective action (BORDENAVE, 1994).

In 1992, Mendes stated that dental education still reproduces retrograde elements such as: the structuring of the course plan in micro-disciplines and dental specialties, the general orientation of the curriculum still directed towards disease, with an emphasis on curative and rehabilitative, educational planning exclusively carried out by teachers and the very nature of teaching staff and research.

Consequently, for dental surgeons to be central to the promotion, protection and recovery of health and the production of humanized care, there is a corollary need for transformations in the process of training these professionals, correcting a mismatch between the orientation of training - still scientific - and the principles, guidelines and needs of the SUS (ALMEIDA and BARA, 2008; BRASIL, 2007; CARVALHO and KRIGER, 2006). Within this concept, Werneck and Lucas, 1996, p.15, add that these desired transformations will require higher education institutions *to "have an enormous need to re-see, re-think and re-create their practices"* (WE R N EC K and LUCAS, 1996, p.15).

Gadotti, 1989; Gonzaga, 1994; Saupe, 1998; Reibnitz, 1998 and Gandin, 1999, among other authors who work with education, recognize Paulo Freire as the pioneer of a liberating pedagogical process. Liberating because knowing is cognizable and also implies a critical awareness of it, and they add that this educator sought to show the political role that education can play, and always plays, in building an open society. This construction, however, cannot be carried out by the dominant elites, who are incapable of providing the basis for a reform policy, but only by the popular masses, who are the only way to bring about change.

Gadotti, Freire and Guimarães, 2000, state that Paulo Freire highlights, in this society of differences, those who oppress and those who are oppressed. He proposes his pedagogy to those who are oppressed, as an itinerary in search of the consciousness of the oppressed class, which harbors within itself the consciousness of the oppressor. Through problematizing education, he seeks the transformation of this reality, through consciousness articulated with challenging and transforming praxis, not without critical dialogue, speech and experience.

The construction of Paulo Freire's Liberating Pedagogical Theory takes us back to an image in which the pedagogical relationship takes place in the interaction between the cognizing subject and the cognizable object. In a relationship in which the educator is a mere interposition between subject and object, but a triple two-way relationship between educator/subject, educator/object and subject/object. In this relationship, the student and the educator refer to the problematization of the object in an attempt to analyze and transform it. As an educator, Freire criticizes the simple transfer of knowledge by non-reflective methods, which shows its superficiality and low retention of knowledge. His focus is on the "teaching-learning-teaching" modalities, leaving the choice flexible depending on the objectives to be pursued (GONZAGA, 1994).

It can be said that the emergence of liberation education brought as a basic assumption that education can and should contribute to a greater process of liberation of the subaltern classes - from the conditions of misery in which they live - since according to Gandin, 1999, p.87, *"education can act in the area of conscientization, that is, in the affirmation of the human being's vocation as a subject"* (GANDIN, 1999, p. 87).

Rezende, 1986, p.166, summarized the guiding principles of Paulo Freire's proposal as follows:

"1- man is the subject of his own education; 2- no one educates anyone; 3- knowledge and ignorance are relative: the content must awaken a new way of relating to life; 4- no one is educated alone; 5- education must take place in man's relationship with his own reality."

For Almeida, 2009, the construction of a reflective educational process with regard to humanization in the work of dentistry is an important strategy for raising awareness, with a view to building a new proposal for health care: humanization. This new knowledge could contribute to a differentiated approach for dental surgeons, with a view to working creatively and providing good quality care, in line with the real needs of the Brazilian population. The same author also added that within this pedagogy, it will be up to the educator to extract the content of reality for learning, providing the possibility of developing an awareness of the social reality of the student. The student is the author of their own knowledge. The educator's role in this methodology is that of a mediator or facilitator, because the educator and the student are the subjects of the act of knowledge. Given these human characteristics, educational action must promote man on this path of discovering himself and not be a mere instrument for adjusting man to the environment - based on this reasoning, we can understand why Freire's proposal is considered a problematizing social theory, since it seeks to relate a new set of information to the student's cognitive structure (ALMEIDA, 2009).

It should also be noted that the choice to work with problematization when introducing the concepts of humanization into dental practice was due to the experience that humanizing practice requires successive approaches, back and forth between the subject and the object of work, with the problematizing methodology becoming an important motivational factor. At this point, the use of this methodology can provide a welcoming environment, stimulating questioning, the identification of problems and, above all, the search for solutions (ALMEIDA, 2009).

To facilitate the operationalization of the problematization assumptions, the entire content of the course "Seminar to Raise Awareness of the Importance of Reception and a Humanized Approach" will go through five steps, in accordance with the problematization arc (BORDENAVE, 1986):

- Observation of reality: the methodology of problematization has as its starting point the observation of reality by the student. Reality is a scenario where various problems can be seen, perceived or deduced and which can be studied together and/or in parts according to the degree of importance attributed to them at the time of observation. This observation of reality is dynamic, i.e. *"depending on the time, space, capacity and/or intentionality of the observers, the problems identified and the relevance attributed to them can be different from one observer to another"* (HORR, 1999, p.124). In addition, the observation of reality depends on the worldview and life experience of the observer, and defines some aspects of why, what and where to observe reality;

- Key points: once the problem has been defined, the important points of the reality observed should be identified. These points are defined as *"key points, they are variables or focuses of the problem situation"* (HORR, 1999, p.127). The identification of these key points is based on the questioning of why or what causes have led to the problem occurring or are related to it;

- Theorizing: after the phase of identifying the key points, comes the

Theorizing, which for Horr, 1999, p.127, is the phase of approaching the truth, during which the following steps are taken:

"the observer asks themselves what they know about the key points, externalizes what they know, listens and acknowledges what others know and the group establishes what additional information they need to seek in order to understand the key points of the chosen problem. It's an internal dialogue that, when shared with the other observers, can generate doubts, questions and concerns, which will give sustainability to generating hypotheses for solutions."

- Hypotheses for solutions: these are the possibilities presented on the basis of theorizing to resolve the difficulty. They must be applicable and feasible to the reality observed, and the application to reality is the application of the strategies chosen to implement the hypotheses;

- Application to reality: According to Horr, 1999, p. 129, *"it can be said that the problem will be solved if there is a change in the observed reality"*, that is, in this context, if the process leads to the transformation of the care provided, becoming more humanized, conscious, providing a therapeutic environment for its users.

3 OBJECTIVES

"... orients the reader to the central purpose of the study and, from there, all other aspects of the research follow (CRESWELL, 2007, p.100)

3 OBJECTIVES

3.1 GENERAL OBJECTIVE

To propose a descriptive analysis of the concepts of humanization of dental practice, through the subject "Seminar to Raise Awareness of the Importance of Reception and a Humanized Approach" applied to the Dentistry course at the Federal University of Juiz de Fora, through a partnership between the latter and the National Program for Reorientation of Professional Training in Health (Pro-Health).

3.2 SPECIFIC OBJECTIVES

- To reorient the process of training future dental surgeons, in order to offer society professionals who are qualified to respond to the needs of the Brazilian population and the operationalization of the SUS;
- Identify and analyse the theoretical and practical content of the discipline relating to humanization;
- Introduce students to social and humanistic practice as early as possible;
- Incorporate a comprehensive approach to the health-disease process into the training process.

4 METHODOLOGY

"It makes no sense to seek scientificity for its own sake, because method is an instrument. It does make sense to do science in order to achieve more favorable objective and subjective conditions for an ever more human history" (DEMO, 1995, p. 260).

4 METHODOLOGY

4.1 CONTEXT

Modern science, in its contradiction, produced knowledge that freed us from the bonds of religious institutions and superstition; however, in the so-called century of enlightenment, with its Cartesian and Newtonian rationalism, it created other dogmas and certainties of a rational nature, diametrically opposed and restrictive to man's understanding (GUERREIRO, 2003, p. 161). It produced the attitude of distancing ourselves from common sense, aesthetic discourse, religious discourse and from understanding what is going on around us, enclosing the scientific process in a system of fixed and maximalist rules, impossible to follow in practice (SANTOS, 1989).

Modern science emerged in the 17th century in opposition to common sense or any form of knowledge - falsoll - and epistemological reflection reached its peak at the end of the 19th century, a period in which industrial society and the spectacular development of technology also emerged and consolidated (SANTOS, 1989). From this perspective, Demo, 1995, states:

"Science is characterized by being a technical instrument, of formal content, with a view to mastering reality, without, however, discussing it. The role of the scientist is to study, research, systematize, theorize, not to intervene, influence or take a position. He portrays, describes, sizes up, but does not propose or oppose, because that would be the stuff of politicians" (DEMO, 1995, p. 23).

In this way, a re-conceptualization of science (a post-modern science) requires epistemology to undergo a hermeneutic reflection, the aim of which is to democratize and deepen practical wisdom (DEMO, 1995, p.248-9). The hermeneutic principle is thus the -understanding of the world of life; it is the understanding that all its parts are determined by the whole, just as the whole is determined by its parts (SANTOS, 1989).

In hermeneutic reflection, the aim is to make scientific knowledge break away from its "leitural code of reality", bringing together other forms of knowledge in the same cognitive field, including common sense itself, an obvious form of knowledge whose protagonists think what exists as it does, have an opinion and think they know what science sets out to know (SANTOS, 1989). From this perspective, Demo (1995, p.18) warns that science is pervaded by common sense because we will never be able to master reality completely, or talk about it with specialized knowledge of all its facets. He understands that common sense, despite being marked by a lack of depth, logical rigour and critical thinking, is also positive because it is knowledge that organizes people's daily lives and, despite being simple, is intelligent and sensitive to the obvious (MATOS, 2006).

From the perspective of this work, which focuses on the concepts of humanization in dental practice, through the discipline - Seminar to Raise Awareness of the Importance of Reception and a Humanized Approach - there are some characteristics of scientificity - thus requiring a methodological approach that is also humanized. From a hermeneutic perspective, the main aim is to understand the possible impact of the concepts introduced and addressed in relation to a phenomenon as human, fragile and sensitive as the ethical-humanist training of a health professional.

Therefore, as Demo (1995, p. 249) said, it is important to look for an appropriate method, "endowed with the humility of those who are willing to listen first, and then speak out, of those who are committed to understanding meanings, significance and values". For this task, it is necessary to balance formal capacity with political perception.

4.2 TYPE OF STUDY

The qualitative approach was chosen as the methodological path, thus ending up in a descriptive, cross-sectional qualitative study that is concerned with a level of reality that cannot be quantified. In other words, according to Minayo et al. in 2002, we worked with the universe of meanings, motives, aspirations, beliefs, values and attitudes, which corresponds to a deeper space of relationships, processes and phenomena that cannot be reduced to the operationalization of variables. The same author also adds that this methodological approach is not concerned with quantification, but with understanding and explaining the dynamics of social relationships, which are the depository of beliefs, values, attitudes and habits. It works with coexistence, with experience, with everyday life and also with understanding structures and institutions as the result of objectified human action - from this point of view: "language, practices and things are inseparable" (MINAYO et al., 2002, p.24).

Qualitative research aims to -provide clarification of a situation so that those being researched become aware of their problems and the conditions that generate them, in order to develop strategic means of resolving themll. It is clear that there is a relationship between reality and the subject, an interdependence between the subject and the object, action and reaction in different situations, since the object of study is not static, making it necessary for the researcher to be inserted in it, in order to make it possible to learn about the meanings that emanate from this experience. The same author insists on the dynamic relationship between subject and object in the process of knowledge. The researcher is an active discoverer of the meaning of actions and relationships that are hidden in social structures (CHIZZOTTI, 1991, p.104).

According to Victora, Knauth and Hassen (2000), the qualitative approach to research is the means used by those who seek to understand the context in which the phenomenon occurs, provides in-depth knowledge of an event and makes it possible to explain behavior.

Minayo and Sanches (1993, p.244) argued that:

"It is in the field of subjectivity and symbolism that the qualitative approach is affirmed. Understanding

human relationships and activities with the meanings that animate them is radically different from grouping phenomena under concepts and/or generic categories given by observations and experiments and by discovering laws that order the social. The qualitative approach brings the subject and the object closer together, since they are both of the same nature; it empathizes with the motives, intentions and projects of the authors, from which actions, structures and relationships become significant".

4.3 METHODOLOGICAL STRATEGY: INSTRUMENTS AND RESEARCH PROCESS

4.3.1 The question

According to Almeida (2007), the great discoveries began with doubt, questioning, or rather, questions, and so they came to fruition - just go back in history and see how they happened.

Today's world provides us with a lot of information - television, books, the internet, magazines, conferences and newspapers - which confuses people because they don't know what questions to answer. We have a generation that is obsessed with answers, but has trouble asking questions. Individuals accumulate data, but have difficulty applying it (ALMEIDA, 2007). According to Alves (2005, p.16) *"Thinking is knowing how to ask questions*". The same author (p.10) also states that *"Our intelligence developed to compensate for our bodily incompetence*".

So where are the valuable questions? And why are so many answers being sought? Nothing replaces the pleasure of discovering. Asking questions is the basis for education. Creswell (2007) stated that in a qualitative study, the researcher should mention the research question, or even questions, and not the objectives or hypotheses. The author goes on to mention the central question:

" [...] is a statement of the question examined in the study in its most general form. The researcher proposes the question, consistent with the emerging methodology of qualitative research, as a general question, so as not to limit the investigation." (CRESWELL, 2007, p.117).

This work began with a question:

- How can the concepts of humanization be introduced into the undergraduate dentistry course through the subject - Seminar to Raise Awareness of the Importance of Reception and a Humanized ApproachH?

Reflecting: there is talk of genomes, cloning, transplants, last-generation drugs, miracle vaccines, in other words, with each passing day the advances in medical science become clear and, in contrast to all this, more diseases are appearing, and even returning. In fact, Maranhâo (2000) states that illness is becoming something common, expected, a natural attribute. Is science heading in the right direction? And if not, what is the reason for so many failures? If health were really so focused on and valued, why are people so sick? According to Rossetti (1999, p. 77), "You don't have to adapt patients to science, you have to adapt science to people", in other words, when you manage to reconcile science and humanization, you will arrive at the much desired health.

This study will not be the absolute answer to the above questions, but will present its experience, through a descriptive analysis, of the introduction of the concepts of humanization in dental practice centered on a compulsory subject in the Dentistry course at the Federal University of Juiz de Fora in partnership with the National Program for the Reorientation of Health Training (PRÓ-Saùde).

4.3.2 Object

The object of the study was a descriptive analysis of the pedagogical content of the subject "Seminar to Raise Awareness of the Importance of Reception and a Humanized Approach" and the practical experience of these concepts through the "Integrated Clinic Internship in Primary Care", which are part of the curriculum of the undergraduate course in Dentistry at the Federal University of Juiz de Fora. The course syllabus is attached (Annex I), as well as the semester plan of activities.

According to Almeida, 2009, the above-mentioned subjects are part of the action plan of the Pró-Saùde project of the UFJF School of Dentistry, which was proposed to introduce students, as early as possible, to a theoretical and practical approach that is more consistent with the real needs of the Brazilian population: actions recommended for primary care in line with the Unified Health System, SUS.

4.3.3 Research subjects and ethical aspects

Qualitative research, according to Creswell (2007, p.188), is described as an interpretative study, where the investigator or subject identifies their personal biases, values and interests in relation to the topic and the research process. Based on the above, it can be said that from a methodological point of view, there is no antagonism between quantitative and qualitative research, as they have different natures: the former works mainly with the data as it is presented and the latter with what the data may represent, incorporating values, attitudes and opinions. Thus, it should be emphasized that qualitative research has the researcher as its main instrument and requires the researcher to maintain close contact with the situation in which the phenomena occur. Thus, the particular circumstances in which a given subject is inserted are essential in order to understand them. In the same way, the people, gestures and words studied must be referenced to the context in which they are produced (BOGDAN and BIKLEN, 1994). It presupposes that the researcher avoids rigid and anticipated definitions, since it is in the research process itself that the research problem is best configured.

Given this methodology, the subject of this study will be the present researcher: Luiz Eduardo de Almeida, an integral member of the creation and execution of the PRÓ-SAÙDE Project at the School of Dentistry of the Federal University of Juiz de Fora, whose attributes in this study are restricted to the development and analysis of all the content covered in the course "Seminar to Raise Awareness of the Importance of Reception and a Humanized Approach", as well as in the "Integrated Clinic Internship in Primary Care".

It should be emphasized that the aim of this investigation was not to test hypotheses; in fact, the use of this dissertation instrument was used as a vehicle to present an experience in permanent health education - after all, the importance of this type of study lies in the possibility for the reader to identify with certain aspects, situations and reflections, in other words, an opportunity for self-analysis based on the other.

With regard to ethical aspects, based on Resolution No. 196⁄96 of the National Health Council, as this research does not involve human beings, since it will only seek descriptive content analysis, it does not need to be assessed by an ethics committee (BRASIL, 1996).

4.3.4 Place of research

This study was carried out at the Faculty of Dentistry of the University

Federal de Juiz de Fora, which is part of the National Program for the Reorientation of Professional Training in Health, PRÓ-SAÙDE, whose action planning is centered on a new curriculum proposal, as described by Almeida (2009, p.30):

"With the new curriculum proposal, it will be possible for students to integrate the knowledge offered by the FO / UFJF Training Institution with the practice of the SUS network services, from a new perspective, starting to understand the service as a place for producing knowledge and a field for stimulating critical reflection on the reality of the population assisted, the challenges and questions, the collective desires, the interdisciplinary work more focused on promoting collective health. In turn, the training institution has the potential to act in a finalistic way in the organization of services. Based on this premise, academics can safely move between places where knowledge is produced and practice scenarios".

4.3.5 . Content analysis

According to the Semester Plan (Annex I), the course "Seminar to Raise Awareness of the Importance of Reception and a Humanized Approach" had a workload of 16 (sixteen) hours distributed over 11 (eleven) theoretical classes. The "Integrated Clinical Internship in Primary Care" was developed in four meetings, with a total workload of 16 (sixteen) hours (Table 1, page 72).

Tabela 1: Conteúdo programático

Módulo teórico – Seminário		
Data	**Descrição**	**Carga horária**
28/08/2009	Apresentação da disciplina	1 hora
04/09/2009	Processo saúde-doença e suas dimensões	1 hora e 30minutos
18/09/2009	Doenças cárie e periodontal: uma percepção holística	1 hora e 30minutos
25/09/2009	Humanização do atendimento odontológico	2 horas
02/10/2009	O SUS no ensino superior (PRÓ-SAÚDE)	2 horas
09/10/2009	Noções de Bioética	1 hora
16/10/2009	Gestão em Odontologia: como planejar, desenvolver e avaliar uma atividade educativo-preventiva (aula 1)	2 horas
23/10/2009	Gestão em Odontologia: como planejar, desenvolver e avaliar uma atividade educativo-preventiva (aula 2)	2 horas
30/10/2009	Apresentação de trabalhos teóricos – Grupos I e II	1 hora
06/11/2009	Apresentação de trabalhos teóricos – Grupos III e IV	1 hora
04/12/2009	Apresentação de trabalhos práticos – Grupos I, II, III e IV (Minimostra) e encerramento	1 hora
	Carga horária total	**16 horas**
Módulo prático – Estágio		
Data	**Descrição**	**Carga horária**
09/11/2009	Estágio Clínica Integrada em Atenção Primária – Grupo I	4 horas
16/11/2009	Estágio Clínica Integrada em Atenção Primária – Grupo II	4 horas
23/11/2009	Estágio Clínica Integrada em Atenção Primária – Grupo III	4 horas
30/11/2009	Estágio Clínica Integrada em Atenção Primária – Grupo IV	4 horas
	Carga horária total	**16 horas**

The descriptive analysis of the subject's content is based on an effort to find a better interpretation of the meanings of the information contained in the aforementioned lessons. The technique chosen was content analysis, as characterized by Bardin (1970, p.42):

"Content analysis is a set of communication analysis techniques aimed at obtaining, through systematic and objective procedures for describing the content of messages, indicators (quantitative or not) that allow the inference of knowledge related to the conditions of production/reception (inferred variables) of these messages."

The same author (1970, p.43-44) presented some fundamental characteristics of content analysis:

- its object is the word, the individual and actual aspect (in act) of language;
- it is an effort to understand the players or the game environment at a given moment, taking into account the meanings (content);
- seeks to know what is behind the words, the other realities through the messages.

As this is a subject that has recently been included in the academic curriculum of the Dentistry course at the Federal University of Juiz de Fora, as well as being aimed at introducing new concepts into dental practice, among the various content analysis techniques presented by Bardin (1970), thematic analysis was chosen because it was considered to be the most coherent with the messages obtained in the classes given, since each topic covered served as a recording unit to study motivations for opinions, attitudes, values, beliefs or tendencies. The author considers this to be one of the easiest, best known and most useful content analysis techniques in a first approach phase.

Content analysis can be said to be a cut that corresponds to meaning and not form, in other words, it is about discovering the nuclei of meaning that appear in the communication - here, in this study, centred on the application of the didactic content mentioned above, emphasizing humanization in dental practice.

In short, based on the methodological references, the analysis was developed following the sequence described:

- Material preparation;
- Data collection;
- Interpretation of results.

In the preparation phase, the subject of the study produced the lecture on the topic to be covered, as well as selecting supporting bibliographic material - in accordance with the syllabus. It is worth noting that all the material was used in accordance with the problematization framework, i.e. by observing reality, identifying the key points, theorizing, hypothesizing solutions and applying them to reality. It should also be noted that all the didactic content will be presented during the discussion of the results.

As far as data collection is concerned, this is a participatory observation study - with the researcher both observing and carrying out the study. It will then be up to the observer to record the information to be analyzed: here focused on the concepts of humanization in dental practice. Bell (2008, p.161) recognizes this:

"Participant observation is not an easy method to carry out or to analyze, but, despite the arguments of its critics, it is a systematic and disciplined study which, if carried out well, helps a lot in understanding human actions and brings with it new ways of looking at the social world."

The interpretation of the results was based on a descriptive analysis of the theoretical content covered, as a way of treating the didactic material applied by the researcher in the course "Seminar to Raise Awareness of the Importance of Reception and a Humanized Approach", extracting its meaning. In order to streamline and standardize the interpretation of the data, we used as a didactic resource the axes of orientation recommended by the National Program for the Reorientation of Professional Training in Health, PRÓ-SAÙDE: Theoretical Orientation, Orientation of Practice and Pedagogical Orientation (BRASIL, 2007, p17).

4.3.6 History

The subject "Seminar to Raise Awareness of the Importance of Reception and a Humanized Approach" was introduced into the academic curriculum of the Dentistry course at the Federal University of Juiz de Fora in the second semester of 2007. As such, the pilot project was carried out during 4 (four) periods of this course, which covers the period from the beginning of this subject until the first semester of 2009.

From these experiments, scientific productions were generated:

- 2009: Presentation - Congress (2ª Reuniâo de Pesquisa Cientifica em Saùde Bucal Coletiva - Unicamp);
- 2009: Award - 1st Place in Panel Presentation (Service Experiences Category) - 2nd Meeting of Scientific Research in Collective Oral Health (Unicamp);
- 2009: Publication - Book (ALMEIDA, 2009);

2009: Publication - Proceedings (PEREIRA et al, 2009a);

- 2009: Publication - Proceedings (PEREIRA et al, 2009b);
- 2009: Publication - Proceedings (ALMEIDA et al, 2009).

It is worth noting that the experience gained from this work served as support for the scenario in which this study was carried out.

4.3.7 Operating scenario

This research refers to a descriptive content analysis of the course "Seminar to Raise Awareness of the Importance of Reception and a Humanized Approach" and the "Integrated Clinical Internship in Primary Care", focusing on the pedagogical content applied in the second semester of 2009, from 28/08/2009 to 04/12/2009.

5 RESULTS AND DISCUSSION

"It's a constant process, involving continuous reflection..." (CRESWELL, 2007, p. 194).

5 RESULTS AND DISCUSSION

As this is a qualitative, descriptive, cross-sectional study, it was decided that both the results and their interpretation and discussion should be included in the same chapter: results and discussion. It should also be noted that, as mentioned in the methodology, in order to streamline and standardize the presentation and interpretation of the data collected, the guidelines recommended by the National Program for the Reorientation of Professional Training in Health, Pró-SAÙDE, were used as an instrument: Theoretical Guidance, Practical Guidance and Pedagogical Guidance, described below.

5.1 theoretical orientation

5.1.1 Reflection

This was followed by the preparation of the theoretical teaching material, which focused on the "political" capacity of the teacher-researcher to offer arguments, through the subject "Seminar to Raise Awareness of the Importance of Reception and a Humanized Approach", which include the ethical-humanistic dimension in the training of dental students at the Federal University of Juiz de Fora.

During the preparation of the theoretical material, doubts began to emerge - confirmed by the following questions: would a professional with a degree in health science, and therefore no specific pedagogical training, be able to teach? Or rather, is it an invasion into someone else's field? Is education restricted to pedagogy?

Carvalho and Kriger (2006, pp.225-226) accurately filled in the gaps in the questions that had hitherto limited this study:

" [...] Pedagogy is at the service of education; it cannot be the exclusive preserve of an enlightened few. Everyone should drink from this fountain. [...] Certainly, specialists are in a better position to carry out pedagogical approaches with greater quality due to their training, which emphasizes specific knowledge of the subject. However, the others simply omit themselves and wait for irretrievable pedagogical precepts, directed from the top down, from the masters of knowledge who have the last word... [...] If that were the case, no one would risk expanding their area of activity. There would be an insurmountable boundary between the activities inherent in the individual's work, according to their specific training, and the rest of science and culture. *[...]* If this were the case, excellent journalists without degrees would be prevented from providing us with their brilliant articles and reports. *[...]* The same would happen with excellent educators, owners of important pedagogical works. They wouldn't venture out (so successfully) into the gardens of Pedagogy. *[...]* Fortunately,

pedagogues are not egotists. On the contrary, they are understanding. They are eager to develop their science and accept everyone's contribution."

We now turn to teaching methodology in the transmission of content - in this study focusing on the lecture. According to Godoy (1988), considered to be the standard technique of traditional teaching, the lecture class has received and still receives a lot of criticism, the most damning of which are: the lack of student participation, the passive receiver in the classroom who is there to absorb the teacher's discourse, and the idea that the class is a homogeneous group in which everyone has the same learning style and the same level of perception.

In contrast to this, Carvalho and Kriger (2006, p.229) presented another side of the lecture:

"[...] When we talk about changes in the conception of teaching, I don't think that the theoretical lesson should simply give way to another technique. Forgetting the past, rejecting the old and fully accepting the new is a radical and simplistic stance. [...] The old theory class is a good working tool, just as the blackboard is practically irreplaceable, even in the face of new teaching aids and resources. [...] After all, the great teachers and thinkers of the past and present were trained in their faculties through lectures, which were the most widespread teaching methodology. [...] Instead of being neglected, it needs to be rethought."

In fact, there's nothing wrong with the lecture, just as there's nothing wrong with any other strategy for transmitting thought - the important thing is to find out when the learning strategy is the best one for achieving certain objectives, and then use it correctly and with adequate prior preparation (CARVALHO and KRIGER, 2006).

Corroborating this, Libâneo (1998) does not discard the lecture and considers it as a means of mobilizing and stimulating the student and in combination with other didactic procedures such as group work and directed study.

In a similar and definitive opinion for this study, Carvalho and Kriger (2006) stated that teaching procedures should be closely related to the teaching objectives, the content to be taught and the students' characteristics and abilities. The best procedure is the one that meets individual or group characteristics. The best teacher is the one who, in each particular situation, knows how to use the most appropriate teaching technique to communicate so that the content can be understood and assimilated without distortion.

Thus, within the aforementioned concepts, for the application of the theoretical content of the course "Seminar for Raising Awareness of the Importance of Reception and Humanized Approach", the expository class was adopted as a didactic instrument for the transmission of content, paying attention to all the arguments explained so far.

5.1.2 Experience

From 28/08/2009 to 23/10/2009, the theoretical module of the SSIAEH course was developed with the 2nd year students of the School of Dentistry at the Federal University of Juiz de Fora. As can be seen in Table 1, page 72, each workshop had its own workload for the teacher-researcher to develop the planned content. The content covered in each lecture will be presented here in descriptive form, as well as the arguments that corroborate their importance in the ethical and humanistic training of dental surgeons.

a. Presentation of the course: 28/08/2009

The content:

The first meeting focused on presenting the course, the chronology of all the content to be covered, as well as the assessment instruments. As can be seen in the lecture, an e-mail was created for the subject, with the aim of bringing teachers and students closer together. As well as making all the theoretical content available, it also acted in the process of active discussion of the subject, in other words, not ending the activities in the classroom.

Based on the idea that introducing or presenting is the way to bring prior information to a job, so that everyone involved understands its role and importance (Creswell, 2007), it can be said that the presentation class achieved these objectives, which favored the entire course of this study.

b. The health-disease process and its dimensions: 04/09/2009

The content:

Seeking a foundation for humanization in health required a deeper and more critical understanding of the health-disease process, considering that this concept must be permanently constructed and correlated to different contexts (ALMEIDA, 2009). This is how the lecture was constructed, the fundamental argumentative basis of which was the essential search for the incorporation of subjective aspects into the illness process. It should be emphasized that at no time did the content neglect scientific rigor; in fact, its most exquisite contribution, and the greatest challenge for health professionals, lies in the call to transform scientific knowledge into true wisdom, more humanized and contextualized with the real needs of the Brazilian population (ALMEIDA, 2009).

The emphasis at this point in the work was on the health-disease process and not just the disease - Rossetti (1999, p. 17) clearly explains the consequences brought about by professionals who were not trained to really work with health:

"We dentists were shown a theoretical science with many scientific bases and in a fragmented way. They showed us muscles, bones, cells, dental materials, bacteria and medicines. They told us what to do with a cavity, a space, what to do with a gum or malocclusion or how to perform surgery. Then we had to put the puzzle heads together and, to do so, we weren't taught how to think, how to decide for ourselves, how to create health in people. We don't know what to do and we do what we've been taught. We restore teeth, close gaps, treat gums, correct malocclusions and perform surgery... However, if you look at your patients, you'll realize that, over time, they'll get sicker and sicker. Health

doesn't grow. On the contrary, illness grows. I've seen beautiful amalgams grow, I've seen them increase in size until they became crowns, three-piece bridges and five-piece bridges; and removable prostheses that have grown all the way to full dentures that continue to grow in height with constant relining... This is because there is an unclear concept of illness and no clear concept of health. As a result, we dedicate ourselves to treating illness rather than creating health. You can never achieve health by treating illness.

We know that the word health has taken on very diverse and even contradictory meanings. The fact is that health and illness do not designate abstract values or absolute situations, nor are they static conditions - obviously change, and not stability, is predominant in life, both from an individual and social point of view (SEGRE and FERRAZ, 1997; BRASIL, 1998).

The lecture highlighted and sought to train the student in a new characterization of health, in search of a broader concept, which requires health professionals to evaluate at least three dimensions: biological, social and psycho-affective - the latter two being rarely valued. The biological dimension clearly appears in the reference to diseases, physiology and pathologies. The social dimension, in the strong reference to the social determinants of the population's health problems, is actually the consequences that the environment can have on an individual. The psycho-affective dimension, in the strong appreciation of the symbolic component and the affective aspects involved in the act of healing and feeling healthy, in other words, self-care. It is with these three dimensions that health professionals must work, discarding the idea of the body as a machine, the dominance of the biological dimension over the others and neglecting the psychological, social and environmental aspects of illness. Understanding the health-disease process as a result of living and working conditions means looking for ways to understand how it rebels in the community. Not only health professionals but also citizens and public institutions must be involved in this effort (SEGRE and FERRAZ, 1997; VALLA, 1982).

In fact, health is a concept to be understood, so health is not taught, it is discussed: the relationship between health and living conditions, the right of the entire population to live in adequate conditions, and so on (COLLARES and MOISÉS, 1989; SEGRE and FERRAZ, 1997). Nevertheless, Alves (2005, p. 82) stated that *"... to educate, to develop the art of thinking..."*.

According to Mendes (1992), dental education still reproduces retrograde elements such as: the structuring of the course plan into micro-disciplines and dental specialties, the general orientation of the curriculum still directed towards the lesion of the disease, with an emphasis on the curative and rehabilitative, the educational planning exclusively carried out by teachers, the nature of teaching staff and research - generating as a corollary the training of highly dehumanized professionals who are poorly prepared for the real health needs of the Brazilian population.

From this perspective, Rossetti (1999, p.24) adds:

" [...] Instead of training doctors to keep the population healthy, they train dentists to keep the

population sick. If, on the contrary, the Faculty was concerned with the health of the population, there would be no subjects for illness and only two for health."

According to Amaral (1991), although the number of colleges has increased over the last two decades in the country, the quality of oral health has not improved. This is because the current teaching model is incapable of providing health care for a large part of the population. University education is very deficient in relation to subjects that deal with social and preventive aspects, often leading to a lack of interest on the part of future professionals. In this sense, adds Alonso (1990), the university must take on the role of reflecting on what it is producing and reproducing as a transforming element with a commitment to society.

According to Valença (1998) and Almeida (2009), educational work based on participation must go beyond the academic training that dental surgeons bring from university, moving towards a more comprehensive understanding of reality. It is from this perspective that dentists should be trained: to become health-promoting agents.

According to Cangussu et al. (2001) and Saliba (2003), health is promoted by ensuring that citizens have decent living conditions, through education, the adoption of healthy lifestyles, the development of individual skills and abilities, the production of a healthy environment, the implementation of public policies aimed at quality of life and health services. The vast majority of the causes of illness and disability could be avoided through preventive actions, provided that these activities were valued and linked to the population. As for curative and assistance measures, aimed at recovering individual health, they should only complement comprehensive health care (ROUQUAYROL, 1993). It is in this scenario that health education in favor of a humanizing practice can play an important role: favoring the process of awareness of the right to health and providing tools for individual and collective intervention in the conditioning factors of the health-disease process (BRASIL, 1998).

Thus, in this context, according to Brasil (2007), for health training, among various concepts, aspects related to the determinants of health and the biological, social and psycho-affective determination of disease should be highlighted, anchored in evidence capable of enabling the critical evaluation of the health-disease process and redirecting protocols and interventions.

Corroborating the above, we can confirm the importance of this topic as an instrument of humanization in health, since it awakens a critical conception in future health professionals regarding the appreciation of the subject as a human being, which is essential for the development of more humanized actions, whether preventive, individual or collective curative, thus contributing to comprehensive care for people and their families. It should also be emphasized that the important thing is to know and recognize that a humanistic approach to the health-disease process reflects a causal perception, i.e. health and disease are not static, isolated states of random causation - one is not healthy or ill by chance. It is a permanent determination, a causal process, which is identified with the way society is organized, or rather, the health-disease process is a particular expression of the general process of social life (ALMEIDA, 2009).

c. Caries and periodontal disease: a holistic view: 09/18/2009

The content:

After working with a broader perception of the health-disease process, it became essential to develop a lecture that would allow for a holistic understanding of the main diseases that affect the oral cavity, thus training professionals who are more capable of a more humanized dentistry that is actually focused on its most important goal: providing the much-desired health. It should also be noted that the theoretical material used problematization as a way of transmitting the content, through an active understanding on the part of the students of the benefits brought about by the holistic and non-reductionist perception of the dental surgeon.

So, first of all, we should clarify the use of the term holism, which is used in various fields of knowledge. One meaning of the term refers to native holism, present in the meanings associated with the praxis of the group of alternative therapists. For them, holism is a set of values applied to therapy that cuts across the dimensions of the medical rationality in which their practice is embedded. In another conception, holism is characterized by a transdisciplinary approach to the construction of knowledge - this area of theorizing directly influences the current transformations in the scientific paradigms of various disciplines, and is more commonly known as complexity science. In it, the terms holistic, complex, systemic and transdisciplinary seem to be used interchangeably, with similar meanings (SOUZA and LUZ, 2009).

In addition to the characterizations mentioned above, there is a third designation for holism, which is the focus of this study, which sees it as a disciplinary category of anthropology, elaborated by Dumont (1985), which characterizes conflicts of values in the macro-social sphere similar to those present in the field of health. The author develops the notion by comparing modern and non-modern societies, distinguishing the latter from the latter by the centrality of the value of man as an individual. Individualism values the individual, neglecting the social totality or subordinating it to man. In order to better understand the meaning of the individual to which the author refers, the opposite category is used: holism values the social totality and neglects the human individual or subordinates it to this totality.

The author also adds that *"the whole is hierarchically superior to the parts because it determines their value and identity"* (DUMONT, 1985, p.255).

It can therefore be seen that the holistic perception offers health professionals, in addition to a modern analysis, a non-reductionist perception of the state of health or illness, and thus directly interferes in the way health professionals develop their practices: integrated and, therefore, more humanized and coherent with the health system in force in Brazil (ALMEIDA, 2009).

In dentistry, it is known that caries and periodontal diseases are the ones that most affect oral health. Within a reductionist perception, different concepts about the etiology of caries have been proposed over time. Ekstrand (2002) provides a historical review of these concepts: he begins with the chemoparasitic theory, stating that various microorganisms in the oral cavity were capable of producing acids through the fermentation of sugar and that they dissolved the hydroxyapatite crystals of the teeth. Later, he defined the term bacterial plaque and isolated streptococci from this plaque when sugar was present in the growth medium. Years later, a specific type of streptococcus was isolated from caries lesions and called Streptococcus mutans. And finally, the classic concept of the three superimposed circles - indicating that the tooth, the microorganisms and the substrate must all be present at the same time for caries to develop (EKSTRAND, 2002).

The term periodontal disease represents a group of pathologies that affect the periodontal tissues: gingivitis and periodontitis. According to Oppermann and Rosing (1997), gingivitis is the most prevalent oral disease. It is found in all ages, as long as plaque accumulates for a certain period of time. The variation that occurs between individuals is due to different host responses.

Brazil is going through an important demographic and epidemiological transition in oral health, with an ageing population and a decline in tooth decay in the younger population, although the phenomenon of polarization persists, with a significant percentage of children and adolescents with a high level of tooth decay. On the other hand, problems linked to traumatic accidents in urban environments, which affect the head, face, mouth and teeth, as well as the occurrence of oral cancer, are becoming increasingly important. What's more, Brazilian adults continue to have the most serious epidemiological legacy, with a large stock of accumulated oral sequelae, especially linked to periodontal diseases and caries, reflected in the rate of edentulism in old age (OPPERMANN and ROSING, 1997; CARVALHO and KRIGER, 2006).

However, the holistic approach to these diseases has completely changed clinical perception and management. For example, caries was only considered when the tooth was cavitated - today it is known that the dental cavity is one of the advanced stages of the disease and that clinically discernible manifestations precede a carious lesion with cavitation. Similarly, periodontal diseases were only noticed when very advanced signs of changes in form and function were detected (OPPERMANN and ROSING, 1997). Therefore, within a holistic dental practice, caries and periodontal diseases are understood as multifactorial infectious-contagious diseases, whose changes in form and function are considered to be their sequelae (ALMEIDA, 2009). In fact, the professional trained in this proposed health intervention must observe and learn the reality of each social space in order to understand the individual, the citizen and the social networks that are built (CORDÓN, 1997).

Within this sample, it can be said that a humanized practice depends a lot on the holistic perception of the health professional, whose job is not to address the patient's illness, but to address the patient. Rossetti (1999, p.77) adds that *"you don't have to adapt patients to science, you have to adapt science to people"*. It has therefore become essential to introduce these concepts into the archaic academic curricula of the dentistry course, so that the future dental surgeon is interested in health and not in disease.

d. Humanizing dental care: 25/09/2009

The content:

For this meeting, a lecture was developed based on the concepts and arguments related to humanization, as well as the benefits brought by a humanized health practice. It should also be noted that the aim of the educational material was much more than to present characterizations and/or designations, but to critically awaken the target audience to a new perspective: the importance and benefits of humanized dentistry.

The concepts of humanization, as well as their perspective on professional training in Dentistry, led us to develop pedagogical material that would stimulate reflection on these concepts among students, here aimed at second-year undergraduates in the Dentistry course. After all, is it possible to teach humanization?

Within this questioning, we considered the need to increasingly deepen the discussion about health within a holistic and humanistic vision, since respect for people's individuality, attentive listening, valuing beliefs and communication, genuine presence, are basic foundations of humanization (ALMEIDA, 2009).

In the experience of this methodology, it was found that the archaic pedagogical curricula, with their mechanistic conception, are dehumanizing, reducing the disease to a merely biological dimension, leading to a greater emphasis on the curative-reparative process, and generating a high-cost practice, low coverage, with little epidemiological impact and inequalities in access (MOYSÉS, 2004; ALMEIDA, 2009).

Therefore, only with the conceptual broadening in the training and practice of professionals in Dentistry was it possible to think of a participatory process of building new meanings, the only way to found a true culture in defense of life, which meets the new challenges of Brazilian dentistry and social demands for more oral health (CARVALHO and KRIGER, 2006; ALMEIDA, 2009).

The humanization proposal faces an immeasurable challenge: that of humanizing health policy and the health system, in a society where so many and such profound forms of injustice and violence prevail in everyday life, the inhumanity of the social determinants of health (GASTALDO, 2005). There can be no humanization project without taking into account the issue of democratizing interpersonal relationships and, as a result, the democracy of health institutions (PUCCINI and CECILIO, 2004; CAMPOS, 2005).

A final warning, as Deslandes (2005) reminds us, the societal proposal of humanization can only be realized if it is taken as a praxis - in the sociological sense of the set of human activities aimed at creating the indispensable conditions for the existence of society, especially in the plane/field of its instituting/instituted practices. It therefore requires perfecting strategies not only for its production, but also for its reproduction. In this sense, investing in the training of professionals with this new awareness is an important strategy, the sustainability of which is based on the dissemination of counter-hegemonic ideological mechanisms and alliances that guarantee adherence and continuous renewal of the proposal (CARVALHO and KRIGER, 2006; BRASIL, 2007; ALMEIDA, 2009).

Thus, the University must provide permanent education, thereby contributing to the consolidation of democratic citizenship. In order to tackle the problems that affect the well-being of the communities in which it operates, it must encourage innovation and transdisciplinarity, by defending and disseminating humanist values in professional training (MOYSÉS et al., 2003).

e. SUS in higher education (Pró-Saùde): 02/10/2009

The content:

Users of the Brazilian public health system often report their experiences questioning the unpreparedness and, above all, the lack of humanization of the health professionals who make up the SUS. With this in mind, the lecture was developed, focusing on the understanding of the doctrinal and organizational principles of the SUS, and centered on awakening the students to the fact that the efficiency and effectiveness of the actions developed by the health system in force in Brazil have a direct relationship with the

training of health professionals, and there is nothing better than offering this as early as possible, that is, during the training of these professionals, which makes it imperative that universities train humanized professionals for the SUS (BRASIL, 2007; ALMEIDA, 2009).

Historically, it is known that the professional training model was aimed at dental care elitist, disconnected from the notion of well-being and quality of life, accessible only to the financial elite of the population - in short, a highly exclusive and totally dehumanized practice, which relegated the development and appreciation of the technician and specialties to the teaching of dentistry (CARVALHO and KRIGER, 2006; BRASIL, 2007; ALMEIDA, 2009).

As a result, dental surgeons were trained to work in the private market - which distanced dentistry from public health policies (ALMEIDA, 2009). The reflection of this sterile dental training was directly reflected in the state of oral health of the Brazilian population, whose public policies for the sector, until the 1990s, acted timidly; after all, until then the understanding of oral health was used in an abstract way, that is, dissociated from the rest of the human body and, in a way, undervalued (CARVALHO and KRIGER, 2006).

In this context, Brazilian dentistry is currently experiencing two types of exclusion: the real exclusion of the population from dental care and the exclusion of a large proportion of newly trained professionals from the job market - an issue that deserves careful consideration by the training units.

It should be noted that the concern with academic training involving technical excellence and social responsibility, which is able to act not only in the treatment of diseases, but also in the promotion of health, dates back to the international strategy of Health for All, from the Declaration of Alma Ata in 1978. Documents in the field of health, foreseeing the dimension that professionals represent in health care, recognize the profound impact that training can have on the quality of the services to be offered to the population, and reinforce the need for a conceptual change in the conception of training. Recognizing that the responsibility for health care does not end with the technical act, but with solving the health problem, is central to the resolubility of the Health System (ADEA, 2004; PLASSCHAERT et al., 2005).

A fragmented curricular structure, whose priority training is technical, without interdisciplinary and multi-professional integration, is what the courses have been offering over time: punctual assistance to patients, perpetuating their stay in the various clinics with little resolution. This difficulty in integrating the curriculum appears in several Brazilian courses (HADDAD et al., 2006).

From this point of view, dentistry is no longer something secondary, but also one of the essential elements of the health system, especially in relation to primary care, and health policies cannot do without oral health since, according to Watt (2005), p.715, *"[...] oral diseases are among the most common chronic diseases, they are important problems for public health because of their prevalence, their impact on individuals and society and the high cost of their treatment'*

The precarious oral health condition of the Brazilian population, as evidenced by epidemiological studies (BRASIL, 2005), the result of years of accumulated and unprioritized needs, is a gap to be addressed in health care in the Brazilian public health system. Thus, according to Almeida (2009), improving access and health levels, reducing the impact of the costs of treating diseases, are essential goals for the system, since access to dental care in the country is still a major marker of social inequalities, or rather, dentistry is one of the important pillars of the dehumanization of the SUS.

Dental surgeons have a fundamental role to play in improving the health conditions of the Brazilian population. However, the professional has been trained according to a model that favors the treatment of diseases, works autonomously, has no experience of teamwork and has little familiarity with the SUS (MORITA and KRIGER, 2004). The lack of articulation between training and health policies is antagonistic to the needs of the population and the consolidation of the SUS (CARVALHO and KRIGER, 2006). It should be stressed that the training of professionals who know, believe in and are committed to the SUS is fundamental to its improvement, generating advances in coverage, efficiency and effectiveness and, consequently, a more humanized system (BRASIL, 2007).

In Brazil, the relationship between dental education and health policies leads us to reflect on two aspects: the growing participation of dental surgeons in public programs, which have become a new job possibility; and the relevance of dental courses in adapting their teaching to a new education that is now playing an important role in public health policies (CARVALHO and KRIGER, 2006; ALMEIDA, 2009).

However, promoting the student's ability to develop intellectually and professionally on an autonomous and permanent basis, enabling them to continue their academic and/or professional training, as well as preparing them to face the challenges posed by the rapid changes in society, the job market and the conditions for professional practice, is now part of the educational process (CARVALHO and KRIGER, 2006; BRASIL, 2007; ALMEIDA, 2009).

In addition, the Curricular Guidelines point to the need to promote, in undergraduate health courses, the articulation between Higher Education and Health, developing skills for health promotion, prevention, recovery and rehabilitation. In this way, the concept of health and the principles and guidelines of the Unified Health System (SUS) are considered fundamental elements to be emphasized (CARVALHO and KRIGER, 2006; BRASIL, 2007; ALMEIDA, 2009).

One of the main actions to stimulate changes in undergraduate courses is the National Program for the Reorientation of Professional Training in Health - PRÓ- SAÙDE. The aim is to support changes in undergraduate courses, bringing higher education institutions closer to the health services, so that the knowledge accumulated in academia can directly influence health practices, while the needs of the health services can also act to broaden the perspective of the vision of social health needs in the academic environment, with regard to both teaching, research and extension. As a result, it is hoped that academic excellence can be combined with social relevance, reflecting directly on better quality health care for the benefit of the Brazilian population (CARVALHO and KRIGER, 2006; BRASIL, 2007; ALMEIDA, 2009).

The bottom line is that training for the SUS, as advocated by the National Curriculum Guidelines, is not about preparing someone for a system that has low

Credibility and is bound to disappear. It's about training professionals to work in the different scenarios of the Brazilian Unified Health System, which is hybrid and must be understood as such. For this reason, professionals need to be trained to work in the public system, in group dentistry, in the management of covenants and accreditations, health plans and even in private practice. Therefore, training for the SUS means training for a complete and complex system, with its own interfaces, which needs to be better studied and understood by the country's higher education institutions (MORITA and KRIGER, 2004; CARVALHO and KRIGER, 2006; ALMEIDA, 2009).

f. Bioethics: 09/10/2009

The content:

Based on the need to introduce humanistic concepts, within an ethical concept, for the training of health professionals, the lecture was developed as part of the theoretical material for the subject "Seminar to Raise Awareness of the Importance of Reception and a Humanized Approach" - the aim was to outline how to think about bioethics and humanization, across the board and in an interdisciplinary way, in undergraduate dentistry, focusing on theoretical discussion and teaching methods.

Bioethics, in its original formulation, was conceived as a new scientific ethic, capable of responding to the deterioration of human-nature relations and whose main objectives would be to guarantee the perpetuation of the human species and of

their quality of life (POTTER, 1970). Over the last 40 years, Ferrer and Alvarez (2005) have stated that bioethics, as a discipline, has acquired different connotations, and variations on the theme can be seen, although it has not ceased to be oriented towards discussing the morality of human acts, as in Kottow's definition (1995, p.53):

"[...] the set of concepts, arguments and norms that ethically value and legitimize human acts, the effects of which profoundly and irreversibly affect living systems, either actually or potentially."

The National Curriculum Guidelines for Undergraduate Dentistry Education (BRASIL, 2002), in its article 4, define, among other requirements:

"[...] Professionals must perform their services to the highest standards of quality and the principles of ethics/bioethics, bearing in mind that the responsibility of health care does not end with the technical act, but with the resolution of the health problem, both on an individual and collective level."

The current transformations experienced in contemporary societies have made bioethics and humanization central themes in medical education (FERREIRA, 2004; REGO, PALACIOS and SCHRAMM, 2004). In a globalized context, with rapidly disseminated information and an increasingly complex science, individuals have to present skills that are different from those usually required, so that there is integration and exercise of a given know-how (SILVA FILHO, 1994; PERRENOUD, 1999).

In fact, aspects such as the extreme speed at which knowledge is produced - and the consequent ephemerality of the truths constructed in scientific know-how (SANTOS, 2003); the need to reorganize health know-how, taking into account integrality, interdisciplinarity and the recovery of the ethical dimension of care/compassion (ZOBOLI and FORTES, 2004); the urgent need to optimize health spending, given the relentless production of knowledge and technological incorporation in health (SANTOS and GERSCHMAN, 2004); the growing questioning traditionally hegemonic values in health practice and the emerging social role of patients and society in general, which have forced a new reflection on the training and practice of professionals in this sector.

(STRUCHINER, GIANELLA and RICCIARDI, 2005); the unequivocal influence of the media and new information technologies on the construction/formatting of man/professional in these early days of the 21st century (STRUCHINER, GIANELLA and RICCIARDI, 2005); the advent/development of control societies - as opposed to the outdated disciplinary societies, built around strategies of confinement (DELEUZE, 1992) - decisively marks the context in which health professionals must be trained, in order to make them capable of responding to the disparate demands of a society in which infectious and parasitic diseases and degenerative diseases are still present (PRATA, 1992; SILVA, PAIM and COSTA, 1999).

Thus, we can see the intertwining of the terms ethics, humanization and education - which can be thought of together, in an articulated and complex way, within the scope of health training, so as to constitute spaces for an interdisciplinary approach - interdisciplinarity understood as "the use of various points of view, but with the cooperative aim of constructing a common theoretical object" (SCHRAMM, 2001, p.38) - and transversal approach. It ends with Almeida (2009), who said that bioethics can be characterized as a bridge between science and humanity, a link between biological knowledge and human values, or even a tool that, through reflection, enables the best possible solution in defense of respect for the person, demanding a humanizing role in health care.

g. Management in Dentistry: how to plan, develop and evaluate an educational-preventive activity: 16/10/2009, 23/10/2009, 30/10/2009, 06/11/2009 and 04/12/2009

The content:

At this point, I'd like to explain the questions that prompted this topic: how can we introduce a humanizing practice to second-year dentistry students at the Federal University of Juiz de Fora? What could they develop within their practical-pedagogical limitations? How could they develop their activities? These questions enabled them to develop collective educational and preventive activities, as well as focusing on the importance of management in these activities.

According to Valença (1998), educational work based on participation must go beyond the academic training that dental surgeons bring from university, moving towards a more comprehensive understanding of reality - from this perspective, dentists should be trained: to become health-promoting agents (ALMEIDA, 2009).

According to Barata (1997), Cangussu et al. (2001) and Saliba (2003), health is promoted by ensuring that citizens have decent living conditions, through education, the adoption of healthy lifestyles, the development of individual skills and abilities, the production of a healthy environment, the implementation of public policies aimed at quality of life and health services. The vast majority of the causes of illness and disability could be avoided through preventive actions, provided that these activities were valued and linked to the population. As for curative and assistance measures, aimed at recovering individual health, they should only complement comprehensive health care (ROUQUAYROL, 1993). It is in this scenario that health education can play an important role: promoting the process of awareness of the right to health and providing tools for individual and collective intervention in the conditioning factors of the health/disease process (BRASIL, 1998).

For Brasil (1998), Aquilante (2003), Garcia (2003), Saliba (2003), Ferreira (2004) and Batista (2005), education and health are closely related and, in particular, health education is the result of the confluence of these two phenomena. In fact, educational action cannot be separated from health action, since the former is implicit in the latter and has objectives and goals based on the health situation of a population, which in turn reflects their living conditions. Education and health should be mutually reinforcing (WHO, 1998; AQUILANTE, 2003; GARCIA, 2003; SALIBA, 2003; FERREIRA, 2004; BATISTA, 2005), since limitations in either are obstacles to the full realization of human potential (MINAYO, HARTZ and BUSS, 2000).

However, the dental surgeon's educational practice, understood as one of the components of basic health actions, is to give people the opportunity to develop a critical conscience, enabling them to take charge of solving their health problems (ROCHA, 1989; VALENÇA, 1998): It is not about telling people what is important to them, but facilitating the conditions for them to see the importance of things (PILON, 1986; VENTURA, 1989; WHO, 1998; AQUILANTE, 2003; GARCIA, 2003; SALIBA, 2003; FERREIRA, 2004; BATISTA, 2005).

Valença (1998), Aquilante (2003), Garcia (2003), Saliba (2003), Ferreira (2004) and Batista (2005) stated that traditional health education, within a hygienist concept, becomes a strange, alienating language, as it tends to be directed towards this or that behavior, forgetting its meaning in the context of the subject's life. When it stops being a process of persuasion or the transfer of education, it becomes a process of empowering individuals and groups to transform reality. In this process, the real participation of those involved must be sought, including the population and health professionals (ROCHA, 1989; WHO, 1998; AQUILANTE, 2003; GARCIA, 2003; SALIBA, 2003; FERREIRA, 2004; BATISTA, 2005).

Health education is a fundamental strategy in the process of forming behaviors that promote and maintain health, because through it it is possible to transform attitudes and behaviors, forming habits in the population the benefit of their own health. Oral health education should be effective in improving individuals' knowledge and, consequently, changing their behavior (WHO, 1998; AQUILANTE, 2003; GARCIA, 2003; SALIBA, 2003; FERREIRA, 2004; BATISTA, 2005).

Educating for health is one of the pillars of health promotion, which aims to empower and give people the opportunity to exercise control and improve their health, and educational actions should be associated with public health policies, clinical actions and community development (PORTILLO, 2000).

However, in order for educational and preventive activities to achieve their objectives, a logical strategy is essential. Corroborating this, Almeida (2009) reports on the importance of planning in health - good ideas are not enough, it is essential to know how to develop the means to make them feasible. Otherwise, possible challenges and threats, which are common, could jeopardize or even make it impossible to carry out major actions. On the contrary, a prepared team will be able, in these situations, to generate strategies and solutions to overcome possible obstacles - showing the importance of health condition management (ALMEIDA, 2009).

Since its inception, health management has gone through successive generations. The first generation consisted of the provision of one or more services, usually care or cure, which were not regularly offered in relation to a particular disease. The second generation moved towards prioritizing actions for the most serious and costly users, a partial response to the law of concentration of severity and health spending. These two generations gave rise to the name disease management, since they were strongly focused on a particular disease, with actions to care for it, cure it or rehabilitate it. The third generation came along with the implementation of health care networks and technology began to cover the entire history of a health condition, through primary, secondary and tertiary prevention measures and with population risk stratification. The fourth generation, which is beginning, is the transformation of disease management into health management or total health management, where the emphasis will be on promotional and preventive measures aimed at optimizing the state of health, with a focus that is less oriented towards curative and rehabilitative measures (MENDES, 2009; COUCH, 1998; ZITTER, 1996).

Thus, Mendes (2009) defined health condition management as the process of managing a specific health condition, already established, through a set of managerial, educational and care interventions, with the aim of achieving good clinical results, reducing risks for professionals and users, contributing to improving the efficiency and quality of health care.

The same author adds that the premise of management is to improve health care throughout the health care network, i.e. the continuum of points of care, and it begins with a correct understanding of the entire history of this condition, expressed in a health condition map (MENDES, 2009).

He also stated that health condition management is a cognitive-intensive process to continuously improve the value of health care and has been considered a radical change in the clinical approach, because it moves from an individual work model, which responds to a patient through curative and rehabilitative procedures, to an approach based on an assigned population, where health conditions are addressed through strategies focused on risk stratification and population-based care (MENDES, 2009).

Thus, 05 meetings were needed to develop this content:

- 16/10/2009:

As can be seen in the lecture (p.141-153), the aim at this point was to train students to develop proper oral hygiene. However, it is known that simply acquiring knowledge is not enough to practise it, and the same happens with brushing (ALMEIDA and PEREIRA, 2010). A second meeting was therefore necessary to highlight the importance of the dental surgeon's role as an educator.

- 23/10/2009:

Rossetti, 1999, p.65, explained:

"... I imagined a brush in the air. A brush in the air does nothing. Behind the brush there has to be a hand; behind that hand there has to be a mind; behind that mind there have to be other minds that stimulate it and these have to have humanistic concepts, concepts of creation, of stimulation for life, not concepts for extraction, for elimination, for disease, for war, for destruction".

- At this point in the course, the lecture was developed (p.153

167) (Annex XV) which dealt with health education and how to plan educational and preventive activities.

- 30/10/2009 e 06/11/2009

o As can be seen in the didactic material applied (p.167-178), these meetings allowed each group to present their respective action plans before they were applied - emphasizing the importance of planning in the efficiency and effectiveness of collective preventive actions (ALMEIDA, 2009).

- 04/12/2009:

o At the last meeting, each group presented their final report (p.179192), covering their experience, focusing on facilities, difficulties, importance, as well as the conclusion of their practical experience at the clinics of the School of Dentistry of the Federal University of Juiz de Fora.

It is also worth noting that a teaching aid was produced, "Knowing and sanitizing my mouth", the aim of which was to make it easier for the students to carry out their practical activities (ALMEIDA and PEREIRA, 2010).

5.2 PRACTICE GUIDELINES

5.2.1 Reflection

After the whole process of theorizing the concepts of humanization with the students of the 2nd period of the Dentistry course at the Federal University of Juiz de Fora, it was time to offer the students the experience and applicability of these concepts, and to this end, the "Integrated Clinic Internship in Primary Care" (Annex I) was developed. This work outlines the principles that guide a proposal for a Supervised Curricular Internship, based on educational goals specific to humanistic content and dental practice.

In this sense, Carvalho and Kriger (2006) state that the Supervised Internship corresponds to the academic activity included in the curricular structure of a course, developed according to the parameters of institutional, legal and pedagogical demands. It is an instrument for integrating students with the socio-economic and cultural reality of the region, based on the professional activity that they will be carrying out. The trainee comes into contact with the different social realities, reflecting on public health practices and policies, the reality of the job market and their own training as an agent for transforming these realities.

Following the approval of the National Curriculum Guidelines (BRASIL, 2002), the Brazilian Dental Education Association (ABENO, 2002) recommended guidelines for supervised internships in dentistry courses. In this report, in addition to recognizing the internship as an instrument for integrating and acquainting students with the social and economic reality their region and the work in their field, it was also stated that this activity should be understood as comprehensive patient care that the dental student provides for the community, both within and outside the classroom (ABENO, 2002).

Almeida (2009) adds that educational practices, those that constitute pedagogical practice in everyday school life, need instruments that can signify the realization of the educational objectives that must have been developed and articulated with the institution's philosophy. One of the important tools for making these practices a reality is the supervised internship - a practical opportunity for students to experience and apply their knowledge, within a logical and real context of how dental practice works.

When students arrive at university, they are faced with theoretical knowledge, i.e. the explanation of reality by renowned researchers. It is often confusing for students to relate theory and practice if they don't experience real moments in which they have to analyze everyday life in the light of the information they have assimilated (BRASIL, 2007; CARVALHO and KRIGER, 2006; ALMEIDA, 2009).

In this way, it is essential to consider that knowledge is built up gradually and implies a constant movement of action-reflection-action on the part of educators, so that an integral formation takes place (CARVALHO and KRIGER, 2006).

And this training takes place through the relationship that is established between theory and practice, based on what the student is able to construct by analyzing reality through the theoretical foundations studied during the course. In this case, the student is the great builder of knowledge and the development of the skills needed to make decisions in the face of the issues we face on a daily basis (CARVALHO and KRIGER, 2006).

"This change of perception, which takes place in the problematization of a concrete reality, in the intertwining of its contradictions, implies a new confrontation between man and his reality. It implies admiring it in its entirety: seeing it from the "inside" and, from that "inside", separating it into its parts and admiring it again, thus gaining a more critical and profound view of his situation in the reality that he does not condition" (FREIRE, 1983, p.60).

Thus, the internship is a privileged moment in which the student positions himself as a scientist and researcher of reality; it is up to him to inquire and question reality, disagreeing with it if it proves to be in opposition to the fundamental issues for the realization of education (CARVALHO and KRIGER, 2006).

The need to improve training leads us to do more research, to carefully analyze conflicts and to reflect that, as trainees, there is still the possibility of not being able to clearly explain the competence that you don't yet have and that you will need to obtain by the end of the course, because when you finish the course, the world of work will look at you as a professional and will demand efficient training from you. Their attitudes will be held to account in relation to their training (CARVALHO and KRIGER, 2006; BRASIL, 2007; ALMEIDA, 2009).

This highlights the need for the student, who will soon be an educator manager, to make a commitment to their holistic education, taking part in classes, guidance and preparing the necessary readings. In other words, understanding knowledge as a value for the ennoblement of the human being (CARVALHO and KRIGER, 2006; BRASIL, 2007; ALMEIDA, 2009).

Therefore, the internship is a time of learning in which you can make mistakes in an attempt to get it right, you can question and question for better training, since, as professionals in the chosen field, appropriate choices and decisions will have to be made (CARVALHO and KRIGER, 2006; BRASIL, 2007; ALMEIDA, 2009). Thus, it is not enough to teach a man a specialty because he will become a usable machine, but not a personality; he needs to acquire a feeling, a practical sense of what is worth undertaking, of what is morally correct (EINSTEIN, 1953).

5.2.2 Experience

a. Integrated Clinical Internship in Primary Care: 09/11/2009, 16/11/2009, 23/11/2009 and 30/11/2009

The National Curriculum Guidelines for Undergraduate Dentistry Courses

advocate that graduates be able to develop a generalist practice of the profession in coherence with the needs of the Brazilian public health system (BRASIL, 2002).

However, there is a clear decontextualization between the practice developed in the teaching clinics of dental schools and the reality of public services, a reflection of a weak teaching-service link that has always depended on the ideological adherence of teachers and students. Extramural teaching and learning activities have always depended more on the voluntariness of the teachers who coordinated them than on institutional support and the participation of the teaching staff as a whole (BRASIL, 2007; ALMEIDA, 2009).

The "Integrated Clinical Internship in Primary Care" (Annex I) was developed as part of the curriculum, with the aim of offering 2nd period students from the Dentistry course at the Federal University of Juiz de Fora, who had completed the theoretical credits covered in the "Seminar to Raise Awareness of the Importance of Reception and a Humanized Approach", a practical experience of the concepts of humanization - after all, the best way to learn is by doing (ALMEIDA, 2009). To this end, the students were divided into four groups, each of which developed an action plan - required during the theoretical module of the SSIAEH - which was developed on previously scheduled dates:

- Group I: 09/11/2009;
- Group II: 16/11/2009;
- Group III: 23/11/2009;
- Group IV: 30/11/2009.

The strategy adopted for this internship was the "Health Training Quadrilateral", which, as described in Brazil (2007b), is:

"explanatory notion of the factors to be considered in the process of permanent health education: teaching practices, care practices, management practices and social control practices in the field of

health".

For a better understanding, the activities carried out by the trainees were divided into four parts, emphasizing that they co-exist:

- <u>Teaching practices:</u>

As has been explained, most higher education institutions still rely on the Flexnerian educational model and, as a result, end up training professionals with an inadequate profile to work within the SUS model, which presupposes Primary Care as the gateway to the health system, where around 80% of the population's health needs are expected to be solved (BRASIL, 2006b; CARVALHO and KRIGER, 2006; BRASIL, 2007).

It was therefore up to the trainees to offer the patients screened by the School of Dentistry of the Federal University of Juiz de Fora educational-preventive activities, emphasizing supervised brushing and, consequently, plaque control - thus acting to prevent, stop, control and even regress the damage caused by caries and periodontal diseases.

The methodology used to introduce the content was the Pedagogy of Problematization, which can be characterized as follows: it begins with the observation of reality, allowing students to express their perceptions, at which point the students select the information and identify the key points of the problem. Once this phase has been completed, theorizing begins, which consists of identifying the causes of the problem observed (CARVALHO and KRIGER, 2006). Here, scientific knowledge helps in the reasoning for understanding the situation. By confronting reality with its theorization, the individual is naturally moved to formulate hypotheses to solve the problem - allowing the use of a double judgment between reality and theory (BRASIL, 2007). According to Piaget, 1973, acquisition is not restricted to just imagining or reproducing a copy of reality, in fact knowing something is done through the ability to act on it.

- <u>Attention practices:</u>

A large part of dental practice in higher education institutions is focused on performing medium and highly complex procedures. Students are often assessed on their ability to perform these procedures. In contrast to all this, primary care, which can solve up to 80% of oral health problems, is rarely, if at all, addressed during the training of these future professionals (BRASIL, 2006b). Thus, it is thought to be extremely important to offer new practice scenarios, adding educational and community facilities to the teaching process, as well as health facilities (CARVALHO and KRIGER, 2006; BRASIL, 2007).

Thus, with the introduction of the "Integrated Clinic Internship in Primary Care", a basic care unit was created, where the student developed both individual and collective care activities. These actions were guided by the following principles: participatory management, access, welcoming, bonding, ethics and professional responsibility. As for the work process, the focus was on interdisciplinarity, comprehensive care, intersectorality, expansion and qualification of care and working conditions. As for the actions, they included Health Promotion and Protection activities (Health Education and Health Prevention) - thus guaranteeing expanded and qualified basic care in line with the needs of the SUS. There was not just one service within the institution, but the creation of lines of care for the users of the services to be provided. In this scenario, the academic became responsible for reception, information, care and referral (reference and counter-reference). In view of this action, the fragmentation of dentistry will leave its long history behind because the disciplines will now be understood as a way of providing comprehensive treatment to patients, improving the quality and humanization of the institution's practices (BRASIL, 2004b).

- Management practices:

Universities still only train dentists to efficiently search for evidence in the diagnosis, care, treatment, prognosis, etiology and prophylaxis of diseases and illnesses - a preparation that is almost entirely restricted to the private market. It is therefore necessary for training institutions to also carry out important innovative initiatives in the area of educational planning and management. And for this to happen, intersectoral links need to be supported and provided, so that permanent health education constitutes spaces for planning, managing and mediating health actions. In this way, services will be provided on the basis of an adequate knowledge of the health reality of each locality in order to create an effectively resolutive practice (BRASIL, 2007).

The aim was to enable university students to plan both individual collective oral health actions. After all, according to Tagliaferro et al. (2005), the initial step in any journey towards a future different from the present must be planning. And planning includes everything from the elaboration to the realization of projects that identify goals, objectives and mechanisms for decision-making and the implementation of actions. Abandoning a normative methodology, which tends to ignore socio-behavioral aspects, and dedicating itself to situational strategic planning, where various actors plan within reality. In this way, it is believed to broaden the professional horizons of the academic, who is no longer just an executor of clinical procedures but has another experience: that of participating as a health manager (TAGLIAFERRO et al., 2005).

- Social control practices:

Social control is a principle and a constitutional guarantee regulated by Law 8142/90 (BRASIL, 1990). This study has a deep identity with the defense of popular participation in health, particularly in adapting health actions to the needs of the population. In fact, the aim was to awaken future health professionals to their role as facilitators and stimulators with the population so that they can exercise their right to participate in defining, executing, monitoring and supervising both individual and collective health actions, moving them from a passive to an active concept, in other words, making them agents of their own health.

5.3 EDUCATIONAL GUIDANCE

5.3.1 Reflection

The reality of the mismatch between what higher education institutions have been training and the type of professional that is needed, imposes changes in the training and work of Brazilian dental surgeons, since work is the central category where different actors from different spaces meet. The necessary changes must begin in professional training and in the worldview reproduced within the academies, because it is certainly in these spaces that the possibilities for the future work of dental surgeons in line with Brazilian needs also begin (BRASIL, 2007; ALMEIDA, 2009).

Thus, with regard to the pedagogical issues related to the concepts of humanization, it should be stressed that the training of the educator becomes a key element, since it is not possible to expect a humanized attitude from the teacher, to the extent that he/she has been prepared to exercise his/her profession only from a technical point of view, as a transmitter of knowledge (CARVALHO and KRIGER, 2006).

Masetto and Prado (2004) state that the role of the educator is to intervene in the learning process with responsibility and commitment; to help the student to take ownership of the knowledge constructed, to give it meaning and to manage differences, to problematize, to motivate, to provoke, in short, to enable the individual to develop their own thinking and discourse.

Almeida (2009) states that, more than in any other position in university teaching, teachers in the health sector need to believe in the merit of their work and the meaning it has for their appreciation of life. In this way, teachers pass it on to their students directly when dealing with patients during clinical procedures. By exemplifying attitudes of respect towards human beings, teachers are able to motivate students towards collective responsibilities in the field of health, and increase their interest in social and human disciplines.

Based on these arguments, it can be said that the teacher can no longer be seen as a monopolizer of knowledge and a transmitter of knowledge, according to the traditional model, but acquires new importance, especially in terms of competence, through the interaction he promotes between educational institutions on the one hand and society as a whole on the other (CARVALHO and KRIGER, 2006; BRASIL, 2007; ALMEIDA, 2009).

Corroborating this, Fernândez (2002) states that innovation is essential in any educational change, but it always involves and has as its reference the teacher. As a phenomenon of change, innovation is subject to modifications produced by the influence of mediators, including the teacher, whose importance is fundamental. Thus, teachers cannot limit themselves to acting in the classroom, but must also seek interaction with their immediate social environment and the general social context. They must be willing to accept change as a constant in their teaching, in the certainty that this attitude is fundamental to the success of innovation. It cannot be stressed enough that innovation processes require teamwork, both in their planning and in their development, an opportunity to awaken the social skills necessary for success in projects of this nature. Finally, the teacher must feel ethically and professionally committed to the process of change, since this process requires the fullest teacher involvement (CARVALHO and KRIGER, 2006).

The adult education process presupposes the use of teaching-learning methodologies that concretely propose challenges to be overcome by the students, that enable them to occupy the place of subjects in the construction of knowledge, participating in the analysis of the very care process in which they are inserted and that place the teacher as a facilitator and guide of this process (BRASIL, 2007).

5.3.2 Experience

Based on the experience of the course "Seminar to Raise Awareness of the Importance of Reception and a Humanized Approach", linked to the "Integrated Clinical Internship in Primary Care", it can be said that this study has achieved its pedagogical success as a cognitive instrument, in terms of raising awareness among 2nd period students at the School of Dentistry of the Federal University of Juiz de Fora of humanistic concepts in dental practice.

Finally, the experiences gained in this work have provided important insights into the importance of ethical and humanistic concepts for the training of academics, by providing an exchange of experiences and by living through the experience, which has led to the emergence of new ideas, new concepts and new directions that contribute to learning.

5.4 INTERPRETING THE RESULTS: "ASK STATISTICS FOR PERMISSION".

Some questions have arisen: how can we evaluate a project developed and based on a qualitative methodology? What procedures should be adopted to evaluate the art of thinking, love or even happiness? After all, it would be impossible, if not ridiculous, to conclude here that someone is 23.46% dehumanized and 76.54% humanized - unfortunately, there are still no multiple choice evaluations and even less the possibility of measuring the humanization of dental practice. Furthermore, Rossetti (1999) adds that the indices that have been used so far are exclusively used to measure illnesses, disregarding social and psycho-affective issues. It would be useful to build indices that assess what has actually been learned. According to Alves (2005, p.72-74):

"What has really been learned is what has survived the purifying action of forgetting. What has been learned is what remains after oblivion has done its work... Only the knowledge that makes sense will remain... Memory keeps what has given pleasure... Memory is intelligent and forgets what doesn't make sense".

As quoted by the WHO (1998, p.11):

"In fact, the teaching-learning process should be constantly evaluated with the participation not only of the project's executors, but also of teachers, parents, students and, if possible, community representatives."

Thus, mathematical values and formulas will not be described here - in fact, one asks for permission from such important statistics. We have opted here for the search for arguments that corroborate the development and applicability of this methodology as an instrument that brings humanistic concepts into dental practice. It is hoped that this study will be a vehicle for reorienting the professional training of dentists, ensuring a comprehensive approach to the health-disease process, promoting transformations in the processes of generating knowledge, teaching and learning and providing services to the population. We close by saying that this study is not about a methodology, or even "a recipe", for humanizing dental practice, after all, it is something to be experienced and not taught.

6 FINAL CONSIDERATIONS

"Not to conclude, but to challenge" (ALMEIDA, 2009).

6 FINAL CONSIDERATIONS

6.1 NOT TO CONCLUDE, BUT TO CHALLENGE...

The starting point of this study was the question of how to introduce humanistic concepts - to students in the 2nd period of Dentistry at the Federal University of Juiz de Fora, through the articulation between the subjects "Seminar to Raise Awareness of the Importance of Reception and a Humanized Approach" and "Integrated Clinical Internship in Primary Care" - as an auxiliary instrument in the construction of a humanized posture in the training of dental surgeons.

Aspects of the human relationship that reflect on behaviour, as well as attitudes considered relevant to the professional attitude and situations that represent humanization in the training of health professionals were surveyed and addressed with the students, through a theoretical approach and a practical contextualization of the humanistic concepts applied. Although this study did not quantify the humanistic potential of the students, it was possible to perceive, through this investigation, a new holistic and progressive attitude, which could help students to reflect on the importance of humanized practice, thus favoring the professional/patient interpersonal relationship - after all, based on all the considerations addressed in this study, humanization can be characterized by the capacity for interaction, or rather, exchange in the relationship between the health professional and their patient.

It is hoped that this study will be a vehicle for reorienting the professional training of dentists, ensuring a comprehensive approach to the health-disease process, promoting transformations in the processes of generating knowledge, teaching and learning and providing services to the population, which requires a pedagogical practice geared towards the emerging paradigms of education, which take a more comprehensive approach to the teaching-learning process, i.e. viewing the student as a complete being, capable of producing knowledge, transforming reality and, when they enter the world of work, perceiving their patient as a human being with biological, social and psycho-affective needs, which need to be met in a holistic way.

The aim of this scientific study was therefore to intervene in the training process: to shift the axis of training, which is still centered on the biological approach, towards more contextualized training that takes into account the social, economic and cultural dimensions of the health/disease process. The main focus of the study was student-population integration, with the consequent inclusion of students in the real practice scenario, with an emphasis on the introduction of humanistic concepts into dental practice - taking into account the training of a qualified professional for the practice of social dentistry, with a generalist, humanistic, critical and reflective vision, with an entrepreneurial and innovative spirit, capable of acting in a multiprofessional, interdisciplinary and transdisciplinary manner, with productivity at the levels of promotion, prevention, treatment and rehabilitation at all levels of health care based on technical-scientific rigor, knowing and understanding the social reality in order to intervene in the oral health problems of the population, based on the ethical and legal principles of the profession.

So, not to conclude, but to challenge, we hope that this study will serve as a stimulus for future work that also sees humanization as a fundamental concept for excellent clinical training for future health professionals. Thus, it can also be said that the course "Seminar to Raise Awareness of the Importance of Reception and a Humanized Approach", linked to the "Integrated Clinical Internship in Primary Care", which is part of the pedagogical project of the School of Dentistry at the Federal University of Juiz de Fora, has served as an important step towards valuing the social aspect of dentistry, which is largely included in the subjects that make up the curriculum and, who knows, perhaps in the future the Department of Social and Collective Dentistry will be structured, dynamic and active, with theoretical and practical subjects throughout the course, reorienting the current curriculum.

7 BIBLIOGRAPHICAL REFERENCES

7 BIBLIOGRAPHICAL REFERENCES

ABBAGNANO, N. **Dicionario de filosofia**. 4 ed. São Paulo: Martins Fontes, 2000. 1232p.

ABENO - BRAZILIAN DENTAL EDUCATION ASSOCIATION. Analysis of the national curriculum guidelines for undergraduate dental courses. **Rev ABENO**. v.1, n.2, p.: 35-38. 2002.

ABRIC, J. C. The structural approach to social representations. In: MOREIRA, A.

S. P.; OLIVEIRA, D. C. (Orgs.). **Estudos interdisciplinares de representaçao social.** 2 ed. Rev. Goiânia/GO: AB, 2000, p. 27-38.

ADEA - AMERICAN DENTAL EDUCATION ASSOCIATION. Competencies for The New Dentist. **Journal Dent. Educ**. v.68, n.7, p.:742-744. 2004

ALMEIDA, L.E. **Oral health: a question of education**. Monograph (Graduation). Federal University of Juiz de Fora, 2007.

ALMEIDA, L.E.; BARA, E.F. **Projeto de Extensao Sabia: a introdução de uma prática integralizadora no ensino odontológico**. Monograph (Specialization). Federal University of Juiz de Fora, 2008.

ALMEIDA, L.E. **PRÓ-SAÙDE: Teaching, Research and Extension**. Juiz de Fora: Editar Editora Associada Ltda, 2009. 256p.

ALMEIDA, L.E; PEREIRA, M.N.; CARMO, A.M.R.; CHAVES, M.G.A.M.; CHAVES- FILHO, H.D.M.; DEVITO, K.L Seminar to raise awareness of the importance of welcoming and a humanized approach: a discipline, a new look. **Journal Ciência e Saùde Coletiva**. Proceedings of the IX Brazilian Congress of Collective Health (ABRASCO). 2009.

ALMEIDA, L.E.; PEREIRA, M.N. **Knowing and sanitizing my mouth**. Juiz de Fora: Editora UFJF, 2010. 40p.

ALONSO, M. E. A. **Current situation of social dentistry teaching in three selected higher education institutions in the state of Rio de Janeiro**. Dissertation (Master's degree in social dentistry). Fluminense Federal University, Rio de Janeiro. 79 p. 1990.

ALVES, R. **Educaçao dos sentidos e mais...** Campinas, SP: Verus Editora, 2005. 126 p.

AMARAL, M. C. P. **Perfil de cirurgiao: dentista do serviço público do municipio do Rio de Janeiro.** Dissertation (Master's Degree in Social Dentistry). Fluminense Federal University, 1991.

AQUILANTE, A. G. The importance of oral health education for preschoolers. **Revista de Odontologia da UNESP**. v.32, n.1, p.: 39-45. 2003.

ARAUJO, M. E. Words and silences in higher education in dentistry. **Ciênc. saùde coletiva**. v.11, n.01. 2006.

BARATA, R. B. Condiçöes de vida e situaçâo de saù saúde. Saùde Movimento, 4. Abrasco. Rio de Janeiro, Baussel R. B. Quality-of-life assessment in outcomes research. **Evaluation & The Health Professions**. v.21, n.2, p.:139-140. 1997.

BARDIN, L. **Content analysis**. Lisbon: 70, 1970. 225p.

BARROS, E. Politica de saù no Brasil: a universalização tardia como possibilidade de construcâo do novo. Rev. **Ciência & Saùde**. v.1, n.1, p.: 05-17. 1996.

BATISTA, R. M. Health education for dental professionals and the population, a path to participation and improved health. **Medcenter: Social and preventive dentistry**. Article. Published December 7, 2005.

Accessed on January 21, 2006. Available at< http://www.odontologia.com.br/artigos.asp?id=597&idesp=12&ler=s>. 2005.

BELL, J. **Projeto de Pesquisa: guia para pesquisadores iniciantes em educaçâo, saù e ciências sociais**. Porto Alegre: Artmed, 2008. 224p.

BENETTON, Luiz Geraldo. **Topics in health psychology:** the professional-patient relationship. Sâo Paulo: L. G. Benetton, 2002. 335 p.

BENEVIDES, R.; PASSOS, E. humanization as a public dimension of health policies. **Ciência & Saùde Coletiva**. v.10, n.3, p.:561-571. 2005a.

BENEVIDES, R.; PASSOS, E. Humanization in Health: a new fad?

Communication, Health, Education. v.09, n.17, p.:389-394. 2005b.

BEZERRA, A.C.B.; PAULA, L.M. A estrutura curricular dos cursos de odontologia no Brasil. **Rev ABENO**. v.1, n.3, pp.: 7-14. 2003.

BOGDAN, R.; BIKLEN, S. **Qualitative research in education: an introduction to theory and methods**. Portugal: Porto, 1994. 336p.

BORDENAVE, J.D. Some pedagogical factors. In: Brazil. Secretariat for Administrative Modernization and Human Resources. **Pedagogical training course for health instructors/supervisors**. Brasilia, 1986, p. 19-26.

BORDENAVE, J.D. In: BRASIL. **Ministério da Saù.** General Coordination of Resource Development for the SUS. Pedagogical Training - Health Area. Reprint of the first edition. Brasilia: MS.,1994,.60p.

BOTAZZO, C. **Da Arte Dentària**. Sâo Paulo: HUCITEC/FAPESP. 2000.

BRAZIL. Ministry of Health. **First National Oral Health Conference**. Brasilia, DF.1986a.

BRAZIL. Ministry of Health. **Final report of the 8th National Health Conference.** Brasilia. 1986b.

BRAZIL. 1988 Constitution. **Constitution of the Federative Republic of Brazil.**

Brasilia, DF, 1988.

BRAZIL. **Laws n°8080 and 8142.** Brasilia: Official Gazette of the Union. 1990.

BRAZIL. Ministry of Health. **II National Oral Health Conference.** Brasilia, DF.1993.

BRAZIL. Ministry of Health. **National Health Council. Resoluçâo 196/96 Diretrizes e Normas Regulamentadoras de Pesquisa em seres humanos.**

Brasilia. Section v.1. p.:21-82. 1996.

BRAZIL. SECRETARIAT OF FUNDAMENTAL EDUCATION. **Parâmetros curriculares nacionais: terceiro e quarto ciclos: apresentaçâo dos temas transversais** / Secretaria de Educaçâo Fundamental. Brasilia: MEC/SEF. p-247-265. 1998.

BRAZIL. Ministry of Education. **Opinion CNE/CES 1300/01.** Brasilia. 2001.

BRAZIL. Ministry of Education. National Education Council. **National Curriculum Guidelines.** Brasilia. 2002.

BRAZIL. Ministry of Health. **Observatory of Human Resources in Health in Brazil: studies and analysis.** (Org) André Falcâo. Rio de Janeiro: FIOCRUZ, 2003.

BRAZIL. Ministry of Health. Executive Secretariat. **Humanizasus - Policy**

National Humanization Program: Humanization as the guiding axis of care and management practices in all instances of the SUS. Brasilia, 2004a.

BRAZIL. Ministry of Health: **Guidelines for the National Oral Health Policy.** Brasilia: Ministry of Health. 2004b

BRAZIL. Ministry of Health. Health Care Secretariat. **SB Brasil 2003 Project: oral health conditions of the Brazilian population 2002-2003: main results.** Brasilia, 2005.

BRAZIL. Ministry of Health. **PNH - National Humanization Policy.** Executive Secretariat. Nùcleo Técnico da Politica Nacional de Humanizaçâo (HumanizaSUS); 2 ed. Brasilia: Ministério da Saùde, 2006a.

BRAZIL. Ministry of Health: **National Health Promotion Policy.** Brasilia: Ministry of Health. 2006b.

BRAZIL. Ministry of Health. Ministry of Education. **National Program for the Reorientation of Professional Training in Health - Pró-Saùde: objectives, implementation and potential development.** Brasilia: Ministry of Health. 2007.88p.

BRAZIL. Ministry of Health. Executive Secretariat. Secretariat for Work Management and Health Education. **Thematic glossary: work management and health education.** Brasilia: Editora do Ministério da Saù. 2007b.

BUSATO, A.L.S.; FERNANDES, C.; GONZALES, P.A.H.; MACEDO, R.P. **Teaching, research and extension in dentistry**. In: Estrela, C. Metodologia cientifica ensino e pesquisa em odontologia. Sâo Paulo: Artes Médicas. 2001. p. 327-45.

BUSS, P M. Health promotion and quality of life. **Rev. Ciência & Saùde**. v.5, n.1, p.: 163-77. 2000.

CAMPOS, R.O. Reflexoes sobre o conceito de humanizaçâo em saù. **Saùde em Debate**. v.27, n.64, p.:123-130. 2003.

CAMPOS, G.W.D.S. Humanizaçâo na saù: Um Projeto em Defesa da Vida? **Interface - Comunicação, Saùde, Educaçao**. v.9, n.17, p.:398-400. 2005.

CANGUSSU, M. C. T.; MAGNAVITA, R.; ROCHA, M. C. B. S. Education and citizenship building in an oral health program in Salvador - BA.

Aboprev Magazine - Living in health. Salvador, v.4, n.1, p.:15-20. 2001.

CARLI, G. **Teacher training and dental education: a perspective under construction**. Master's thesis (Postgraduate Diploma in Dentistry).

Lutheran University of Brazil, 2007.

CARVALHO, A.C.P.; KRIGER, L. **Dental Education**. Sâo Paulo: Artes Médicas, 2006. 264p.

CHIZZOTTI, A. **Pesquisa em ciências humanas e sociais**. Sâo Paulo: Cortez, 1991. 165p.

COLLARES, C. A. L.; MOISÉS M. A. A. Educaçâo , Saù e Formaçâo da Cidadania. **Education and Society**. Sâo Paulo. 10 (32). 1989.

CORDÓN, J. The construction of an agenda for collective oral health. **Cadernos de Saùblica**. v.13, n.3. 1997.

COUCH, J.B. **Desease management: na overview** - In: COUCH, J.B. (Editor) - The health-care professional's guide to disease management: patient-centered care for the 21st century. Gaithersburgh, Aspen Publication, 1998.

CRESWELL, J.W. **Research design: qualitative, quantitative and mixed methods**. 2 ed. Porto Alegre: Artmed, 2007. 248p.

CRUZ. E.A. **Pràticas Profissionais dos Trabalhadores em Central de Maternidade e Esterilizaçâo: representaçoes sociais da equipe de enfermagem.** Doctoral Thesis, Federal University of Ceará, Fortaleza, Ceara-Brazil, 2003.

DELEUZE, G. **Post-scriptum on control societies**. In: Deleuze G. Conversations, p.:1972-1990. Rio de Janeiro: Editora. p.34. 1992.

DEMO, P. **Metodologia cientifica em ciências sociais**. 3.ed.. Sâo Paulo: Atlas, 1995. 293p.

DESLANDES, S.F. O Projeto Ético-Politico da Humanização: Conceitos, Métodos e Identidade. **Interface - Comunicação, Saùde, Educaçâo**. v.9, n.17, p.: 401-403. 2005.

DUMONT, L. **O individualismo: uma perspectiva antropológica da ideologia moderna**. Rio de Janeiro: Rocco. 1985.

EINSTEIN, A. **How I see the world**. Sâo Paulo: Nova Fronteira. 1953.

EKSTRAND, K. Diagnosis of tooth decay. In: BUISCH, I. P. Promoting oral health in the dental clinic. Sâo Paulo: Artes Médicas, p.125-147. 2002.

FERNANDEZ, J.T. **The innovative teacher.** In: De La torre S, Barrios O. Curso de formaçâo para Educadores. Sâo Paulo: Madras Editora. 2002.

FERREIRA, A.B. H. **Novo Aurélio século XXI. O dicionàrio da lingua portuguesa**. 3 Ed. Rio de Janeiro: Nova Fronteira, 1999.

FERREIRA, N.S.C. Repensando e ressignificando a gestão democràtica da educação na -cultura globalizadall. **Educ Soc**. v.25, n.89, p.:1227-1249. 2004.

FERRER, J.J.; ALVAREZ, J.C. **Para fundamentar a bioética**. São Paulo: Loyola; 2005.

FOULQUIÉ, P **Dicionàrio da lingua pedagògica**. Portugal: Livros Horizonte, 1971.

FREIRE, P. **Educaçâo e Mudança**. Rio de Janeiro: Editora Paz e Terra. 1983.

FREITAS, S.F.T. **História Social da Càrie Dentària**. Bauru: EDUSC. 2001.

GADOTTI, M. **Invitation to read Paulo Freire** . Sâo Paulo: Scipione, 1989. 175p.

GADOTTI, M.; FREIRE, P.; GUIMARAES, S.. **Pedagogy: Dialogue and Conflict**. 4th ed., Sâo Paulo: Cortez, 2000. 127p.

GANDIN, D. **Planejamento: como pràtica educativa.** Sâo Paulo: Ed. Loyola, 1999. 111p.

GARCIA, P. P. N. S. Oral Health Knowledge in Schoolchildren: Effect of a Self-Instruction Method. **Revista de Odontologia da UNESP.** V.33, n.1, p.: 41-46. 2003.

GASTALDO, D. Humanization as a Conflicting, Collective and Contextual Process. **Interface - Communication, Health, Education**. v.9, n.17, p.:395-397. 2005

GODOY, A.S. **Didatica para o ensino superior**. Sâo Paulo: Editora Iglu. 1988.

GOFFMAN, E. **Stigma: notes on the manipulation of damaged identity**. 4ª Ed. Rio de Janeiro: Editora Guanabara Koogan. 1988.

GONZAGA, A.A.. **Popular Health Manual: from allowing disease to collective and dialogical actions in health**. Master's Degree Dissertation (Post-Graduation in Nursing). Federal University of Santa Catarina, 1994.

GRANT, Valerie. Making room for medical humanities. **Méd. Humanit**. v. 28, n. 1, p.: 45-48. 2002.

GUERREIRO, L. **Education and the sacred**: the therapeutic action of the educator. Rio de Janeiro: Lucena, 2003. 96p.

HADDAD, A.E.; LAGANA, D.C.; ASSIS, E.Q.; MORITA, M.C.; TOLEDO, O.A.;

RODE, S.M.; FERREIRA, S.H.; FERREIRA, S.L.M. **Contribuiçâo das avaliaçôes do MEC na identifcaçâo da coerência dos projetos pedagógicos do curso de graduaçâo em odontologia às diretrizes curriculares nacionais.** Brasilia: INEP/EC. P.:119-152. 2006.

HARRISON, R.L.; WONG, T. An oral health promotion program for an urban minority population of preschool children. **Community Dent. Oral Epidemiol**. v.31, n.5: p.392-399. 2003.

HEIDEGGER, M. **Conferences and philosophical writings**. Sâo Paulo: Abril Cultural, 1979.
IBAMA, **History of the Environment.** 2006. Consulted at http://www.ibama.gov.br/institucional/historia/index.htm . Accessed on 09/11/2006.

HORR, L. Building the Arc of Problematization. In: **Education, work and nursing**. Florianópolis: Universidade Federal de Santa Catarina, 1999. p.124137.

HOUAISS, Antonio; VILLAR, Mauro de Salles; FRANCO, Francisco Manoel de Mello. **Dicionario Houaiss de lexicografia.** Rio de Janeiro: Objetiva, 2001.

IYDA, M. **Saúde Bucal: uma pràtica social**. In: Ciências Sociais e Saùde Bucal: Questoes e Perspectivas (C. Botazzo & S.F.T de Freitas org.). Bauru, Sâo Paulo: EDUSC/UNESP. p.127-139. 1998.

JODELET, D. Social Representations: an expanding field. In JODELET, D. (org). **Social Representations.** Rio de Janeiro: UERJ, 2001.

KOTTOW, M. **Introdución a la Bioética**. Santiago: Universitària; 1995.

KRIGER L. **Changes in professional training: the efforts underway**.

Available at: http://www.universidadesaudavel.com.br/. Accessed on: 06 Jun 2005.

LALANDE, A. **Vocabulario tècnico e critico da filosofia**. 3 ed. Sâo Paulo: Martins Fontes, 1999. 1336p.

LÉVITAS, E. **Humanism of the other man**. Petrópolis. Editora Vozes, 1993.

LIBÂNEO, J.C. **Didatica**. 16ª reprint. Sâo Paulo: Cortez, 1998.

LUCAS, S.D. **Professional training of dental surgeons graduating from two higher education courses with different orientations**. Dissertation - Faculty of Education, UFMG, Belo Horizonte, 1995.

LUCIETTO, D.A. **Percepções dos docentes e reflexões sobre o processo de formaçao dos estudantes de Odontologia**. Dissertation (Master's Degree in Public Health). Oswaldo Cruz Foundation, 2005.

LUZURIAGA, L. **Diccionario de Pedagogia**. Buenos Aires: Editorial Losada S.A. 1960.

MAGALHAES, R. Monitoring social inequalities in health: meanings and potential of information sources. **Ciênc. saùde coletiva**. v.12, n. 3. 2007. Available at:< http://www.scielo.br/scielo.php?script=sci arttext&pid=S1413-81232007000300016&lng=en&nrm=iso>. Accessed on: 26 Oct 2007.

MARANHAO, D.G. Caring for the link between health and education. **Cad. Pesqui**. [online]. 2000, no. 111 [cited 2006-11-27], pp. 115-133. Available at: <http://www.scielo.br/scielo.php?script=sci arttext&pid=S0100-15742000000300006&lng=pt&nrm=iso>. ISSN 0100-1574. doi: 10.1590/S0100-15742000000300006. 2000.

MARCOS, B. **Pontos de epidemiologia**. Belo Horizonte: ABOMG. 1984.

MASETTO, M.T.; PRADO, A.S. Learning evaluation process in a Dentistry course. **Rev. ABENO**. V.4, n.1, p.:48-56. 2004.

MATOS, P.E.S.; TOMITA, N.E. The inclusion of oral health in the Family Health Program: from the university to the training centers. **Cad Saùde Pùblica**. v.20, n.6, p.: 1-11. 2005.

MATOS, M.S. **An analysis of the students' profile and the ethical-humanistic dimension in the training of dental surgeons in two dental courses in Bahia**. Thesis (Doctorate). Federal University of Bahia, Faculty of Education, 2006.

MELO, J.J.P. **O estado romano e a formaçao do cidadão, Teoria e pràtica da educaçao.** 2005. http://www.dtp.uem.br/rtpe/volumes/v8n3/completos/008.pdf. Accessed on 15/07/2007.

MENDES, E.V. **The production of knowledge for dental practice in Latin America**. Paper presented at the First Conference of Dental Schools and Faculties in Latin America, Faculty of Medical Sciences, Autonomous University of Santo Domingo, October 12-16, 1980. mimeogr. Apud PRETO, S.M. A odontologia no SUS: o desafio da pràtica integral. 1991. Dissertation (Master's degree in social dentistry). Fluminense Federal University, 1992.

MENDES, E.V. **Health care networks.** Belo Horizonte: ESP-MG. 2009.

MENEZES, J. D. V.; LORETTO, N. R. M. **Abeno: 50 years of contribution to Brazilian dental education**. Maringà: Dental Press. 2006. p.: 27-40.

MINAYO, M.C.S.; SANCHES, O. Quantitative-qualitative: opposition or complementarity? **Cad. Saùde Pùblica**. v. 9, n. 3, p. 237-48. 1993.

MINAYO, M. C. S.; HARTZ, Z. M. A.; BUSS, P. M. Quality of life and health: a necessary debate. **Ciênc. saùde coletiva**. [online]. 2000, vol. 5, no. 1 [cited 200611-28], pp. 7-18. Available from: <http://www.scielo.br/scielo.php?script=sci arttext&pid=S1413-81232000000100002&lng=en&nrm=iso>. ISSN 1413-8123. doi: 10.1590/S1413-

81232000000100002. 2000.

MINAYO, M.C.S. **Pesquisa Social: teoria, método e criatividade**. 21.ed.. Rio de Janeiro: Vozes, 2002. 80p.

MOLINA, A. **Humanizaçâo da assistência à saù: bases teórico-filosóficas e sugeroes pragmàticas.** (2002). http://www.crmmt.cfm.org.br/jornal/jonais 2002/Dezembro/pag_8 htm. Accessed on 15/07/2007.

MOREIRA, T. P.; NATIONS, M. K.; ALVES, M. S. C. F. **Teeth of inequality: oral marks of the experience lived in poverty by the community of Dendê, Fortaleza, Ceará, Brazil**. Cad. Saùde Pùblica, Rio de Janeiro, v. 23, n. 6, 2007 . Available at:< http://www.scielo.br/scielo.php?script=sci arttext&pid=S0102- 311X2007000600013&lng=en&nrm=iso>. Accessed on: 26 Oct 2007.

MORITA, M.C.; KRIGER, L. Changes in Dentistry courses and the interaction with SUS. **Revista da ABENO**.v V.4, n.1, p.:17-21. 2004.

MOSCOVICI, S. **Representações Sociais: teoria e pràtica.** 2 ed. Joâo Pessoa: Editora Universitària/ UFPB, 2003.

MOYSÉS, S.J. The humanization of education in Dentistry. **Pro-Posiçôes**. v. 14, n. 1, p.: 87-106. 2003.

MOYSÉS, S.T.; MOYSÉS, S.J.; KRIGER, L. Humanizing Education in Dentistry. **Rev. Abeno**. v.3, n. 1, p.:58-64. 2003.

MOYSÉS, S.J. Health policies and the training of human resources in dentistry. **Rev ABENO**. V.1, n.4, p.: 30-37. 2004.

NARVAI, P.C. **Human Resources for Oral Health Promotion**. In: ABOPREV: Promoçâo de Saùde Bucal (L. Kriger org.). Sâo Paulo: Editora Artes Médicas. 1999. pp.448-463.

NORONHA, A B. Graduation: change is needed - transformations depend on education and health policies. **Radis Comunicação em Saùde**. v.5, p.:9-16. 2002.

OPPERMANN, R. V.; ROSING, C. K. **Prevention and treatment of periodontal diseases**. In: KRIGER, L. (Org.) ABOPREV: oral health promotion. Sâo Paulo: Artes Médicas, p.255-281.1997.

WORLD HEALTH ORGANIZATION, O. M. S. Health-promoting schools: A healthy environment and better health for future generations. Communication for Health No. 13, **Pan American Sanitary Bureau, Regional Department of the WHO,** translated by Renata Ferreira e Ferreira. Washington, D.C. Print version. p. 1-19. 1998.

PAIM, J. S. **Health care in Brazil**. In: Brazil, Ministry of Health. Health in Brazil - contributions to the agenda of research priorities. Brasilia, DF. 2004. p:15-44.

PEARCE, W B. New communication models and metaphors: the shift from theory to practice, from objectivism to social constructionism and representation. In: SHNITMIAN, D.F. (org). **New**

paradigms, culture and subjectivity. Translated by Jussara Hambert Rodrigues. Porto Alegre: Artes Médicas, 1996. p. 172-183.

PEREIRA, M.N. **Effectiveness of person-centered learning in the training of professional dentists**. Master's dissertation. Juiz de Fora: Higher Education Center; 2000.

PEREIRA, M.N.; ALMEIDA, L.E.; CARMO, A.M.R.; DEVITO, K.L.; SANTOS, A.P.M.; OLIVEIRA, M. Seminar to the sensibilization of the importance of sheltering and humanized services: a subject, a new look. **Brazilian Journal of Oral Sciences**. v.-, n-, p.:50-51. 2009a.

PEREIRA, M.N.; ALMEIDA, L.E.; CHAVES, M.G.A.M.; CHAVES-FILHO, H.D.M.; DEVITO, K.L.; SOUZA, T.S.; REIS, W.C.F.B.; RODRIGUES, C.M. Seminàrio para sensibilização da importância do acolhimento e enfoque humanizada: uma disciplina, um novo olhar. **Brazilian Oral Research**. v.3, s.1, p.:329. 2009b.

PÉRET, A.C.A. **Public policies in higher education and health and the training of dental teachers in a critical dimension**. Doctoral thesis. Belo Horizonte: Federal University of Minas Gerais; 2005.

PERRENOUD, P. **Building Competencies from School**. Porto Alegre: Artmed; 1999.

PESSINI, L.; PEREIRA, L.L.; ZAHER, V.L.; SILVA, M.J.P Humanization in health: the rescue of being scientific competence. **Mundo Saùde**. v.27, n.2, p.: 203-205. 2003.

PESSOTTI, I. The humanistic formation of the doctor. **Medicina**. v.-, n. 29, p.: 440-448. 1996.

PIAGET, J. **Language and thought in the child**. Rio de Janeiro: Fundo de Cultura. 110p. 1973.

PILON, A. F. The development of health education: an updating of concepts. **Rev. Saùde Pùblica**. [online]. 1986, vol. 20, no. 5 [cited 2006-11-28], pp. 391-396.

Available at:< http://www.scielo.br/scielo.php?script=sci arttext&pid=S0034-89101986000500009&lng=en&nrm=iso>. ISSN 0034-8910. doi: 10.1590/S0034-89101986000500009. 1986.

PINTO, V. G. **Saùde Bucal Coletiva**. Sâo Paulo: Editora Santos. 2000.

PIZZATTO, E.; GARBIN, C.A.S.; GARBIN, A.J.Î.; SALIBA, N.A. O papel do professor no ensino odontológico. **Rev Saùde Debate**. v.28, n.66, p.: 52-57. 2004.

PLASSCHAERT, A.J.M.; HOLBROOK, W.P.; DELAP, E.; MARTINEZ, C.;

WALMSLEY, A.D. Profile and Competences for the European Dentist. **Eur. J. Dent. Educ**. v.9, p.:98-107. 2005.

PORTILLO, J. A. C.; PAES, A M. C. Self-perception of oral health-related quality of life. **Rev Bras. de Odont. em Saùde Coletiva**. V.1, n.1, p.: 75-88. 2000.

POTTER, V.R. Bioethics, science of survival. **Biol Med**. v.14, p.:173-153. 1970.

PRATA, P.R. The epidemiological transition in Brazil. **Cad. Saùde Pùblica**. v.8, n.2, p.:168-175. 1992

PUCCINI, P.D.T.; CECILIO, L.C.D.O. The humanization of services and the Right to Health. **Cadernos de Saùde Pùblica**. v.20, n.5, p.:1342-1353. 2004.

REGO, S.T.A.; PALACIOS, M.; SCHRAMM, F.R. **The teaching of bioethics in undergraduate health courses**. In: Marins JJN, Rego S, Lampert JB, Araùjo JGC.

Medical education in transformation: instruments for the construction of new realities. São Paulo: Hucitec; Rio de Janeiro: Brazilian Association of Medical Education; 2004.

REIBNITZ, K.S. Enfermagem: espaço curricular e processo criativo. In: SAUPE, R.

Nursing Education: from the constructed reality to the possibility under construction. Florianópolis: EDUFSC, 1998, p.187-218.

REZENDE, A.L.M. **Saùde: dialética do pensar e do saber**. Sâo Paulo: Carez, 1986. 160p.

RIZZOTTO, M.L.F. As Politicas de Saù e a Humanizaçâo da Assistência. **Revista Brasileira de Enfermagem**. v.55, n.2, p.:196-199. 2002.

ROCHA, C.M.V. **Educaçao em saùde: breve histórico e perspectivas**. In: BRAZIL. Ministry of Health. Coletânea educaçâo, saùde e educaçâo em saùde.

Brasilia, DF, 1989.

RODRIGUES, J. C. **O tabu do corpo**. Rio de Janeiro: Editora Achiamé; 1979.

ROGERS, C. R. **Client-Centered Therapy**. São Paulo: Martins Fontes, 1992.

ROSA, W A. G.; LABATE, R. C. Programa Saùde da Familia: a construção de um novo modelo de assistência. **Rev. Latino-am Enfermagem**. v.13, n.6, p.: 1027-34. 2005.

ROSSETTI, H. **Saúde para a Odontologia**. 2 ed. Sâo Paulo: Editora Santos, 1999. 146 p.

ROUQUAYROL, M. Z. **Epidemiology & Health**. Epidemiology, Natural History and Disease Prevention. In: Rouquayrol, M. Z. 4ª edição. Rio de Janeiro: MEDSI. p. 7-22. 1993.

SALIBA, N. A. Oral health education program: the experience of the Araçatuba School of Dentistry -UNESP. **Rev. Odontologia Clin.-Cientif**. Recife, V.2, n.3, p.:197-200. 2003.

SANTOS, B.S. **Introduçao a uma ciência pós-moderna.** Rio de Janeiro: Graal, 1989. 176p.

SANTOS, B.S. **A discourse on the sciences**. Sâo Paulo: Cortez. 2003.

SANTOS, M.A.B.; GERSCHMAN, S. The segmentation of the supply of health services in Brazil: institutional arrangements, creditors, payers and providers. **Ciênc.**

Saùde Coletiva. v.9, n3, p.:795-806. 2004.

SANTOS, J. F.; WESTPHAL, M. F. Emerging practices of a new health paradigm: the role of the university. **Rev. Estudos Avançados**. v.13, n.35, p.: 71-87. 1999.

SAUPE, R. (Org.) **Nursing Education: from the constructed reality to the possibility under construction**. Florianópolis: Federal University of Santa Catarina, 1998. 101p.

SCHAFF, Adam. **The computer society:** the social consequences of the second industrial revolution. 4.ed. Sâo Paulo: Brasiliense, 1995. 157p.

SCHRAMM, F.R. **The different approaches to bioethics**. In: Palâcios M, Martins A, Pegoraro OA. Ethics, science and health: challenges for bioethics. Petrópolis: Vozes. p.2845. 2001.

SECCO, L.G.; PEREIRA, M.L.T. Concepôes de qualidade de ensino dos Coordenadores de graduaçâo: uma análisis dos cursos de odontologia do Estado de Sâo Paulo. **Interface - Comum Saùde Educ**. v.8, n.15, p.: 313-330. 2004.

SEGRE, M; FERRAZ, F.C. The concept of health. Rev. Saùde Pùblica. V.31, n.5, p.:538-42. 1997.

SILVA FILHO, H.P. **O Empresariado e a Educaçâo**. In: Ferreti CJ et al. (org.) New technologies, work and education. A multidisciplinary debate. Petrópolis: Vozes; 1994.

SILVA, L.M.V.; PAIM, J.S.; COSTA, M.C.N. Inequalities in mortality, space and social strata. **Rev Saùde Pùblica**. v.33, n.2, p.:187-197. 1999.

SOUSA, M.F. **Os sinais vermelhos do PSF**. Sâo Paulo: HUCITEC, 2002.

SOUZA, E.F.A.A.; LUZ, M.T. Bases socioculturais das pràticas terapêuticas alternativas. **História, Ciôncias, Saùde**. v.16, n.2, p.393-405. 2009.

STRUCHINER, M.; GIANELLA, T.R.; RICCIARDI, R.M.V. **New Information Technologies and Health Education in the face of the Communication and Information Revolution**. In: Minayo MCS, Coimbra Jr. Criticas e Actuantes: ciências sociais e humanas em saù na América Latina. Rio de Janeiro: FIOCRUZ, p. 257-272. 2005.

STRUCHINER, M.; VIEIRA, A.R.; RICCIARDI, R.M.V. Analysis of knowledge and conceptions about oral health of dental students: evaluation through concept maps. **Cad. Saùde Pùblica**. v.15, n.2, p.:1-15. 2005.

TAGLIAFERRO, E. P. S.; TENGAN, C.; KASSAWARA, A. B. C.; FONSECA, D. A.

V.; PEREIRA, A. C.; MENEGHIM, M. C. **Strategic planning in oral health in the city of Piracicaba, SP:** A **case study**. Arquivos em Odontologia: 41(4): 273-368. 2005

TOLEDO, L.C.M. **Humanizaçâo do edificio hospitalar, um tema em aberto.** (2007). http: //mtarquitetura.com.br/HUMANIZAÇÂO_%20 EDIFICIO_HOSPITALAR.pdf. Accessed on 15/07/2007.

VALENÇA, A. M. G. A **Educaçâo em Saù na Formaçâo do Cirurgiâ-Dentista: da necessidade à pràtica participativa.** Niterói: Editora UFF, 1998.

VALLA, W. Education, health and citizenship: scientific research and popular advice. **Cadernos de saùblica**. Rio de Janeiro. V.1, n.8, p.:30-40. 1982.

VENTURA D. V. R. **Participatory action as an educational practice in leprosy control**. In: Brasil. Ministry of Health. Coletânea educaçâo, saù e educaçâo em saù. Brasilia, DF, 1989.

ViCTORA C.G.; KNAUTH, D.R.; HASSEN, M.N.A. **Qualitative research in health: an introduction to the theme**. Porto Alegre: Tomo Editorial, 2000. 136p.

WATT, R.G. Strategies and approaches in oral disease prevention and health promotion. **Bulletin of The World Health Organization**. v.83, n.9, p.:711-718. 2005.

WERNECK, M.A.F.; LUCAS, S.D. Supervised internship: an experience of oral health teaching/service integration. **Arq.Cent. Est. Curs. Odont.** V. 32, n. 22, 1996.

WEYNE, S. C. **The Construction of the Health Promotion Paradigm - a Challenge for the New Generations**. In: ABOPREV: promoçâo de saùde bucal / coordination by Léo Kriger. 2ª edição. Sâo Paulo: Artes Médicas. 1999. p. 01- 26.

WOLF, S. M. R. The psychological meaning of tooth loss in adult subjects. **Rev Assoc Paul Cir Dent**. v.52, p.:307-15. 1998.

ZANETTI, C.H.G. **Odontologia: habilidades e escolhas**. 2001. Available at: <http:www.saudebucalcoletiva.unb.br>. Accessed on: June 2004.

ZITTER, M. **A new paradigm in health care delivery: disease management**.

In: TODD, W.E.; NASH,D. (Editors) - Disease management: a systems approach to improving patient outcomes. Chicago, American Hospital Publishing Co. 1996.

ZOBOLI, E.L.C.P.; FORTES, P.A.C. Bioética e atençâo bàsica: um perfil dos problemas éticos vividos pelos enfermeiros e médicos do Programa de Saùde da Familia, Sâo Paulo, Brasil. **Cad Saùde Pùblica**. v.20, n.6, p.:1690-1699. 2004.

8 ANNEXES

8 ANNEXES

Annex I: Syllabus for the subjects "Seminar to Raise Awareness of the Importance of Reception and a Humanized Approach" and "Integrated Clinical Internship in Primary Care".

SIX-MONTH ACTIVITY PLAN

2ND SEMESTER 2009

- Seminar to Raise Awareness of the Importance of Reception and a Humanized Approach - Preparation for Entry to the Integrated Clinical Internship in Primary Care (ORE 030T).

-Integrated Clinical Internship in Primary Care (STG 010A and STG 010B).

1- IDENTIFICATION

Federal University of Juiz de Fora - School of Dentistry:

- Departments:

Social and Children's Dentistry (OSI);

Restorative Dentistry (ORE).

- Subjects:

○ Seminar to raise awareness of the importance of welcoming and a humanized approach - Preparation for entry to the integrated clinic internship in primary care (ORE 030T);

Integrated Clinical Internship in Primary Care (STG 010-A and STG 010B).

- Responsible:

Advisor: Professor Marilia Nalon Pereira;

Master's student: Luiz Eduardo de Almeida.

- Target population: students enrolled in the 2nd period of Dentistry.
- Workload: 50 min/class

Timetable: STG 010-A and STG 010-B - Mondays from 2 p.m. to 6 p.m. (Practical content);

ORE 030-T - Fridays, from 12 noon to 1 p.m. (theoretical content).

2- SUMMARY

In partnership with the National Program for the Reorientation of Health Professionals (PRÓ-SAÙDE), the courses - Seminar to raise awareness of the importance of welcoming and the humanized approach - preparation for entry to the internship in integrated primary care (class ORE030, T) and -Integrated Clinic Internship in Primary Care (classes STG010-A and STG010-B) were proposed in order to provide the student-intern with a theoretical and practical approach to the actions recommended by the Unified Health System (SUS) for user care at the primary level, in the oral health care service.

3- OBJECTIVES

3.1. General objective:

- Reorient the training process for health professionals in order to offer society professionals who are qualified to respond to the needs of the Brazilian population and the operationalization of the SUS.

3.2. Specific objectives:

- Incorporate a comprehensive approach to the health-disease process and health promotion into the training process in the health sector;
- Offering students a more comprehensive understanding of reality;
- Introduce students as early as possible to the practical world of their profession.

4- SCHEDULED ACTIVITIES

1) Seminar to raise awareness of the importance of welcoming and a humanized approach - Preparation for entry to the integrated clinic internship in primary care.

a.Strategy:

- Teaching practices - Compulsory subject

To introduce academics to theoretical content that is rarely or not at all covered during their undergraduate studies: PRÓ-SAÙDE; Health-disease process and its dimensions; Hygiene techniques and self-care of the mouth; The SUS (Unified Health System) is everyone's problem; The humanization of dental care; Creation of a questionnaire to measure the satisfaction of those served by the dental clinics of the Faculty of Dentistry / UFJF.

It should be noted that the methodology to be used to introduce the content described above will be the Pedagogy of Problematization, which can be characterized as follows: it begins with observing reality, allowing students to express their perceptions - at this point the students select the information and identify the key points of the problem. Once this phase has been completed, theorizing begins, which consists of identifying the causes of the problem observed. Here, scientific knowledge aids reasoning in order to understand its theoretical principles. Confronting reality with its theorization, the individual is naturally moved to formulate hypotheses to solve the problem - allowing the use of a double judgment between reality and theory. After all, acquisition is not restricted to imagining or reproducing a copy of reality, in fact knowing something is done through the ability to act on it.

b. Development:

The course lasts 16 hours, divided into meetings:

- 1st meeting (28/08/2009): Presentation of the course;
- 2nd meeting (04/09/2009): The health-disease process and its dimensions;
- 3rd meeting (18/09/2009): Caries and periodontal diseases: a holistic perception;
- 4th meeting (25/09/2009): Humanization of dental care;
- 5th meeting (02/10/2009): SUS in higher education (PRÓ-SAÙDE);
- 6th meeting (09/10/2009): Notions of Bioethics;
- 7th meeting (16/10/2009): Management in Dentistry: how to plan, develop and evaluate an educational-preventive activity (class 1);
- 8th meeting (23/10/2009): Management in Dentistry: how to plan, develop and evaluate an educational-preventive activity (class 2);
- 9th meeting (30/10/2009): Presentation of theoretical work - Groups I and II;
- 10th meeting (06/11/2009): Presentation of theoretical work - Groups III and IV;
- 11th meeting (04/12/2009): Presentation of practical work - Groups I, II, III and IV (IIª Minimostra) and closing.

II) Integrated Clinical Internship in Primary Care.

a. Strategy:

- Attention practices:

A large part of dental practice in higher education institutions is geared towards performing medium and highly complex procedures, and students are often assessed on their ability to perform them. In contrast to all this, primary care, which can solve up to 80% of oral health problems, is little or even not addressed during the training of these future professionals. It is therefore extremely important to offer students new practice scenarios, adding educational and community facilities to the teaching process, as well as health facilities.

As for the actions, they will include Health Promotion and Protection activities (Health Education and Supervised Oral Hygiene).

- Social control practices:

Social control is a constitutional principle and guarantee regulated by Law 8142/90. This study has a deep identity with the defense of popular participation in health, particularly in adapting health actions to the needs of the population. In fact, the aim is to train health professionals as facilitators and stimulators with the population so that they can exercise their right to participate in defining, executing, monitoring and supervising both individual and collective health actions, moving them from a passive to an active concept, in other words, making them agents of their own health.

b. Development:

The students will be divided into four groups, each of which will be responsible for attending a clinic, through the following actions:

- Creation and realization of a lecture on oral health to be given in the waiting room for patients to be assisted by the clinics of the Faculty of Dentistry/UFJF;
- Supervised brushing in the brushing room;
- Application of a questionnaire, created by the group, aimed at evaluating the satisfaction of those served with the service offered by the institution;
- Presentation of work related to the content applied.

5- STRATEGY

- Entrepreneurial education.

It can be said that education and entrepreneurship merge into a singular, broader and more integrative experience. In its conception, an entrepreneur is someone who independently provides for his or her own livelihood. It is someone who offers positive value to the community.

In fact, in active/entrepreneurial educational methodologies, the student is understood as a person who has an important cognitive-affective background, as well as an underlying culture that identifies them with a contextualized reality. The teacher's role is to point out ways in which the student can continue their education, acting as a mediator, problematizing the situations they experience in their daily lives and training spaces. In this methodology, the higher education institution is not confined to its physical space, and there is a diversification of possibilities for educational scenarios, as well as their actors.

6- EVALUATION PROCESS

1) Seminar to raise awareness of the importance of welcoming and a humanized approach - Preparation for entry to the integrated clinic internship in primary care.

- Attendance: 10 points.
- Evaluation of meetings: 90 points

- Health-disease process and its dimensions: 10 points;
- The humanization of dental care: 10 points;

- SUS is everyone's problem: 10 points;
- Bioethics: 10 points;
- Development and applicability of the Questionnaire: 15 points;
- Development and application of a collective activity: 15 points.
- Presentation of final work (Mini-Sample): 20 points.

- Total: 100 points.

II) Integrated Clinical Internship in Primary Care.

- Attendance: compulsory;
- Evaluation of conduct within the clinic:
- Total: 100 points.

7- BIBLIOGRAPHICAL REFERENCES

ALMEIDA, L. E. **Seminar to raise awareness of the importance of welcoming and a humanized approach: preparation for entry to the integrated clinic internship in Primary Care**.

PRÓ-SAÚDE: Project of the Faculty of Dentistry/UFJF. Juiz de Fora: 2007. 46p.

8- SCHEDULE

DATE	SCHEDULE	TEACHER	CONTENT
28/08/2009	13:00 to 17:00	Luiz Eduardo	**Theoretical:** -Presentation.
04/09/2009	13:00 to 17:00	Luiz Eduardo	**Theoretical:** - The health-disease process and its dimensions.
18/09/2009	13:00 to 17:00	Luiz Eduardo	**Theoretical:** - Caries and periodontal diseases: a holistic view.
25/09/2009	13:00 to 17:00	Luiz Eduardo	**Theoretical:** - Humanization in dental care. - Film
02/10/2009	13:00 to 17:00	Luiz Eduardo	**Theoretical:** - The Unified Health System in higher education (PRÓ-SAÙDE).
09/10/2009	13:00 to 17:00	Luiz Eduardo Aline Spagnol	**Theoretical:** - Notions of Bioethics.
16/10/2009	13:00 to 17:00	Luiz Eduardo	**Theoretical:** - Management in Dentistry: how to plan, develop and evaluate an educational-preventive activity (lesson 1).

23/10/2009	13:00 to 17:00	Luiz Eduardo	**Theoretical:** - Management in Dentistry: how to plan, develop and evaluate an educational-preventive activity (lesson 2)
30/10/2009	13:00 to 17:00	Luiz Eduardo	**Theoretical:** -Presentation of the questionnaire and the activities to be carried out - Groups I and II.
06/11/2009	13:00 to 17:00	Luiz Eduardo	**Theoretical:** -Presentation of the questionnaire and the activities to be carried out - Groups III and IV.
09/11/2009	13:00 to 17:00	Luiz Eduardo Aline Spagnol Karina L. Devito	**Internship:** Group I (10 academics) - Sanitizing techniques; -Application of the satisfaction questionnaire.
16/11/2009	13:00 to 17:00	Luiz Eduardo Aline Spagnol Karina L. Devito	**Internship:** Group II (10 academics) - Sanitizing techniques; -Application of the satisfaction questionnaire.
23/11/2009	13:00 to 17:00	Luiz Eduardo Aline Spagnol Karina L. Devito	**Internship:** Group III (10 academics) - Sanitizing techniques; - Application of the satisfaction questionnaire.
30/11/2009	13:00 to 17:00	Luiz Eduardo Aline Spagnol Karina L. Devito	**Internship:** Group IV (10 academics) - Sanitizing techniques; - Application of the satisfaction questionnaire.
04/12/2009	13:00 to 17:00	Aline Spagnol Karina L. Devito Luiz Eduardo	**Theoretical:** -Final work presentation - Groups I, II, III and IV.

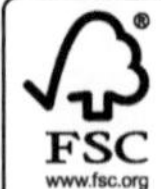

MIX
Papier aus verantwortungsvollen Quellen
Paper from responsible sources
FSC® C105338

Printed by Books on Demand GmbH, Norderstedt / Germany